Assess Your True Risk
of Breast Cancer

Patricia T. Kelly, Ph.D.

Assess Your *True Risk of* BREAST CANCER

An Owl Book
Henry Holt and Company
New York

Henry Holt and Company, LLC
Publishers since 1866
115 West 18th Strteet
New York, New York 10011

Henry Holt® is a registered trademark of
Henry Holt and Company, LLC.

Library of Congress Cataloging-in-Publication Data

Kelly, Patricia T., date.
Assess your true risk of breast cancer / Patricia T. Kelly.—1st ed.
p. cm.
"An Owl book."
Includes index.
ISBN 0-8050-6468-0 (pbk.)
1. Breast—Cancer—Risk factors.   I. Title

RC280.B8 K448   2000   00-044851
616.99'449—dc21

Henry Holt books are available for special promotions
and premiums. For details contact: Director, Special Markets.

First Edition 2000

Printed in the United States of America

1   3   5   7   9   10   8   6   4   2

Contents

Acknowledgments

I have been helped by many wonderful people in the course of developing this book. Jill Kneerim, my agent, offered encouragement and essential, timely, practical assistance from the very start. I am deeply grateful for her thoughtful, professional, and knowledgeable approach. I remain indebted to Dr. Susan Love for introducing me to her. Caroline Pincus's expertise, feedback, and perceptive comments helped me to shape the book and present its material in a manner that felt increasingly direct and accessible.

Deborah Brody, my editor at Henry Holt and Company, provided meaningful editorial help. I feel fortunate to have had the benefit of her editorial eye.

I am particularly grateful to friends and colleagues for discussions about and review of some of the material. The thoughtful comments and suggestions of John C. Arpels, M.D., Elliott Foucar, M.D., Lynn Godmilow, M.S.W., William H. Hindle, M.D., Michael D. Lagios, M.D., and Rodger Shepherd, M.D., M.P.H., helped to improve the accuracy and clarity of the book. Any remaining mistakes or oversights that remain are mine.

I am indebted to librarians Peggy Tahir, Marianne Zaremska, and Nancy Phelps for their expertise and unwavering support. Judy Feld provided encouragement for the project throughout as well as astute strategic support. Eric O. Gold, M.S., used his considerable creative talents to help me develop the book's figures, then carefully prepared them for optimal reproduction. I feel fortunate to have had his help. Timothy A. Donlon, Ph.D., graciously provided photographs of the chromosomes used in two of the figures.

Sid Gershgoren critically yet lovingly reviewed large parts of the book and remained robustly cheerful and encouraging throughout. With his help, the process was largely joyful.

I especially thank the many patients I have seen over the years who shared their hopes, concerns, and questions with me. In so doing, they taught me a great deal—not only about how to present risk information—but also about what truly matters in life. For their gift, and for the many friends and colleagues who have encouraged and sustained my quest to provide clear, useful information and help to individuals concerned about cancer risk, I am truly grateful.

Assess Your True Risk
of Breast Cancer

Introduction

Whether two, five, or fifty women get together, you often hear about breast cancer risks: what's recently been reported to increase risk, decrease risk, or even prevent breast cancer. And you hear how these latest reports contradict those of only a few months or years ago. There's a great deal of new information, lots to talk about, but little or no clarity or help for a woman who is trying to use the information to make decisions. Generally, conversations reflect women's uncertainties about what their breast cancer risks actually are, what the risks mean, and what to do about them. For example, you may hear:

- "Why are the breast cancer risks higher in my area than elsewhere?"
- "Did you see the article about fat/alcohol/having a child after age 30 and how it increases/doesn't increase breast cancer risk?"
- "I've heard that hormone replacement therapy may be good for my heart and will help me think more clearly and get some sleep, but then I worry about taking hormones with my family history."
- "I read that genetic testing won't be helpful, but my cousin is being tested and says her doctor thinks I should be, too."
- "My doctor doesn't seem to be enthusiastic about my taking tamoxifen, even though I've read that it reduces breast cancer risk."
- "I've seen three different doctors and I *still* can't figure out what my breast cancer risk is now that I have this diagnosis of ductal carcinoma

in situ. She says it's a precancer, but I wonder how she can tell that it hasn't already spread."
- "Since I have a high breast cancer risk, I wonder what to do now."

If you have questions and concerns like these, you are not alone. Most women *are* uncertain about what their breast cancer risk actually is, which parts of the constantly changing information they can trust, and what to do about an increased risk. This book is designed to give you a clear, useful understanding about what your breast cancer risks really are—not the same endlessly repeated statistics that leave you bewildered, but solid, dependable information that actually makes sense. In addition, I'll provide tools to help you evaluate the importance and relevance of risks. These tools will be useful in assessing the information you read here and for making decisions about study results that will be reported in the future. With information about how to assess risks, you will be able to evaluate information in a meaningful context and will be able to determine *what this information means for you and your unique life situation*—in other words, what to do with the risk information once you understand its relevance.

Who Will Benefit from This Book?

⚘ If you have wondered what your breast cancer risks really are, and would like specifics instead of generalizations, this book is for you. It is for you if you are looking for information that will enable you to make informed decisions about your breast health care. It is also for you if you think that:

- You have heard enough about breast cancer risk and are concerned that more information will only lead to more confusion in your life.
- You won't be able to analyze statistics, since numbers are not your strong suit.
- Risk information has little meaning since you either will or won't be diagnosed with breast cancer.
- Reading and thinking more about cancer risk won't be good for your emotional health.
- Reading about breast cancer will make you feel more isolated and alone.

If you have any of these thoughts, please read on! I will discuss each of them to show you that this book *is* for you as well.

You may think you've heard enough about breast cancer risk and that more information will only lead to more confusion and uncertainty. Actually, you are more likely to be confused if you have too little relevant information, too much extraneous information, or if you lack access to a broad framework into which various facts can be placed to help you make sense of the whole. The information in this book is simple, direct, and to the point. It covers the latest study results and shows you how to evaluate their relevance to you.

Even if you have read a great deal about breast cancer risks, you may find that much in this book is new and surprising. For example:

- The familiar "1 in 9" statistic, understood in proper context, actually means that the average woman's breast cancer risk is just 2% to age 50, 6% from 50 to 70, and 3% from 70 to 85.
- The breast cancer rate for women up to age 50 has hardly changed since 1973.
- Most women who have both a mother and sister with breast cancer will never be diagnosed with breast cancer themselves. The risk to this group, to age 69, is about 16%.
- An increased hereditary risk of breast cancer can be passed through your father's side of the family as well as your mother's.
- The much publicized 30% to 50% increase in breast cancer risk to women who take hormones at menopause means in absolute or "real" numerical terms only *0.6 more cases of breast cancer per 100 women* from ages 50 to 70.
- Only 5% to 10% of breast cancers are strongly hereditary.
- Most women who have benign breast disease (also called fibrocystic breast disease) are not at increased risk of breast cancer.
- Ductal carcinoma in situ, the type of "breast cancer" with the greatest rate increase in recent years, lacks the biological capacity to metastasize or spread to other parts of the body.
- A woman who started her first period at a young age, who started menopause at an older age, or who never had a child has a risk of breast cancer that is very slightly increased, if at all, compared to women with other reproductive histories.
- In the much-publicized study announcing a 49% reduction in breast

cancer risk to high-risk women who took tamoxifen, breast cancer risk was actually reduced by *only* 1.8 cases of breast cancer *per hundred women* over a period of nearly six years.
- Women whose relatives have postmenopausal, not just premenopausal, breast cancer, may be at increased breast cancer risk due to strong hereditary factors.
- A risk may be reported as "statistically significant" and still be quite small.
- In some circumstances, when genetic testing finds no mutation that increases cancer risk, a woman may still have a high breast cancer risk due to hereditary factors.

Some of these statements may seem contradictory, impossible, or just plain wrong. However, once you learn how to assess risk and interpret the results of studies, a process that uses a few commonsense tools and simple rules, you will appreciate more fully that risks and statistics need to be put in context if they are to be useful—and how you can do this.

You may think you won't be able to analyze statistics, since numbers are not your strong suit. In this book you will find that common sense, in conjunction with some very simple guidelines and tools, will allow you to determine when a risk figure is likely to have relevance to you and when it may be misleading. For example, if you hear about a 50% increase in risk, you will know to go on to look for more useful and meaningful statistics.

From the material you will read in the chapters to come, you will be able to judge for yourself how important a risk may be. Barbara*—one of my patients whose mother, sister, and aunt had all been diagnosed with breast cancer—said rather exultantly when she understood these approaches to risk: "Now I feel free!" She was talking about freedom from the worry and uncertainty she had previously endured each time a new study about breast cancer risk appeared. My great wish is that this book will do the same for you.

You may think that risk information can have little or no meaning to you personally, since you either will or will not get breast cancer. This

---

*Not her real name. Here and elsewhere I have changed the name and other aspects of a situation to protect the privacy of the individual; any similarity to a person or family is due to chance and entirely unintentional.

book will show you how to put your breast cancer risk into perspective so that you can live more peacefully with it. The information presented here will better equip you to make informed breast health care decisions that can help to protect your life and improve its quality. You will then come to view breast cancer risk in much the same way as other risks in your life—and will be able to take the necessary steps to be and feel as safe as possible.

You may think that reading and thinking about cancer risk won't be good for your emotional health. Breast cancer risk can be an uncomfortable topic, so you may wonder how dwelling on it will help. This book will show you (or remind you) that when a troubling aspect of life is ignored, feelings about it can grow strangely and vigorously. At times they can crop up in painful and unexpected ways and even diminish the quality of your life—for example, by draining your energy or creating anxiety about cancer risk when you hear the latest media report. However, once you have learned how best to safeguard your health and have more information about how to design the most appropriate breast health program, you can begin to take steps to lessen any uncomfortable feelings about breast cancer. As you do, you may find that your feelings about breast cancer risk change, and, even more, you will probably find they have lost their power to unexpectedly intrude on your life. In time, they can just melt away, like a block of ice exposed to the sun.

You may feel isolated, alone, or singled out due to your experiences with a loved one's breast cancer. This book will show you that many other women have experienced similar, if not identical, feelings when their friends and relatives had breast cancer. By hearing about others' experiences, you may feel less alone and better able to cope with your own reactions to cancer risk.

How This Book Came to Be

For twenty years I have practiced as a medical geneticist, specializing in providing information about breast and other cancer risks to women of many different ages and in many different circumstances. Some were diagnosed with cancer, some had friends or relatives with cancer, while others did not. All were, however, interested in learning about their own breast cancer risks, so they could do what was necessary to be as safe as possible and to feel safe. As my patient Barbara said:

> When my friends ask if it's scary for me to come and see you, I tell them I was much more scared before I understood my risks and what I could do about them. This is the best thing I've done in a long time for me. Remember how lost I felt when I first came? Now I feel safe because I've had a chance to decide what's right for me—and I'm doing it!

Many women, like Barbara, live with great concern and even fear about their breast cancer risk. They recalculate their risks each time new information becomes available. They agonize over diet and fret about the age they were when they started having periods. They think back to the age when their first child was born, and feel even worse if they haven't had a child. And they remain unclear about the meaning of these risks or are misinformed about how large or small these different risks actually are. Some multiply the various risks, others add them together. As you will see, neither approach is supported by scientific findings. Many women tell me that they have read and heard so much contradictory information that they are no longer sure what to believe or even whether it's worth trying to continue to understand. The result for many is a nagging anxiety.

In the last twenty years thousands of women have shared with me their experiences regarding cancer and cancer risks. I've heard their questions, their concerns, their misunderstandings, their fears and hopes, and their ways of coping—not only their own but also those of their family and friends. Over time, with their help, I learned about the type of information that enabled them to take control of their breast health care decisions, responsibly and with assurance. In this book I transmit to you not only risk information but also what these brave and resourceful women have taught me about how they learned to live more comfortably with risk and how they made peace with uncomfortable and even frightening past experiences.

This book will provide you with clear, specific, useful information about hereditary and nonhereditary breast cancer risks—the same type of information that has been so useful to my patients. You will learn simple, commonsense ways of evaluating risks, using the approaches I have developed for my patients over the years. Without having to take a course in statistics, you will learn to apply rules that will make it possible for you to avoid confusion in the future and to move forward with security.

Throughout the book I will tell you about individuals like Barbara, who have come to me seeking information and have in the process taught me a great deal about the kinds of information they need and the techniques they use to help themselves live more comfortably with their risk. I think you will find that these approaches and examples will help you also.

Just as I did for Barbara, I want to answer your questions and provide you with the information that will help you make decisions that are right for you. I also want to help you achieve the settled peace of mind that comes from realizing that you *do* have options and that you have learned the steps to take to protect yourself. My aim is to help you reach decisions that are appropriate for *you*. I think you will find, as many of my patients have, that the news about breast cancer risk and survival after a breast cancer diagnosis is far better than you may have heard and that more options are available than might be apparent.

Again and again women tell me that one of their greatest concerns is that they won't hear about important information or that they will fail to grasp its importance. They don't want to blame themselves in the future for either what they did or did not do to protect their health. This is a valid concern, since risk information often comes densely packaged and can be expressed in an insider's code. Because the information is compressed, a woman can think that she understands it and may even repeat what she knows to her doctors, leading them to believe also that she understands it. Later, she may discover that she did not fully grasp the implications or the ramifications of the information, sometimes with sad consequences. In this book, I will "unpack" the material and will spell out its ramifications. Once you see how it is done, you will be able to do it yourself.

The Organization of the Book

I've presented the information in this book in approximately the same sequence and in the same manner as I do in my office. The book is divided into three sections. Part I, "The Human Part," deals with the powerful and frequently long-lasting emotions that often arise when a woman has a friend or relative with breast cancer. Part II contains information about some of the more frequently discussed breast cancer risks. Here I present information and tools for assessing what these risks actually mean to an individual. You will need the information in these chapters to make informed decisions about your breast health care program. The material in Part III is designed to help you make use of the factual information in Part II.

You will find some repetition in the chapters to remind you of important points raised previously. When appropriate, I will refer you to an earlier chapter's information if it will help to make the section you are reading clearer. At the end of each chapter you will find a list of "Key Points to Remember." These are a summary of the most important topics in that chapter. In the Notes section you will find complete citations for studies discussed in each chapter.

Chapter 1 focuses on some of the normal reactions many women have when a friend or relative is diagnosed with breast cancer. The women I see are frequently abashed or even embarrassed by the strength of their concern about breast cancer or the way it remains as a nagging worry at the back of their minds. Some say that their feelings about breast cancer are "irrational" or "unreasonable." To me, however, their concerns and their reactions are quite understandable and result from factors such as these:

- Increased mass media reporting about breast cancer risks, which makes it difficult for women to escape hearing about the topic.
- Increased public discussion by women who have been diagnosed with breast cancer, leading to wider circles of women who hear about their experiences.
- Risk information that is frequently presented in formats that are not relevant or useful to an individual woman.
- Little or no information about how to assess the magnitude or importance of a particular breast cancer risk or to know when a woman has taken appropriate steps to safeguard her health.
- Lack of information about the normal emotional consequences to a woman when a friend or relative is diagnosed with breast cancer.

Women who have a friend or relative with breast cancer, a group that is largely forgotten, may be strongly influenced by a loved one's breast cancer, even years later. Many have not had a chance to discuss or explore their experiences or the feelings that arose during and after that time.

Those of you who have a friend or relative with breast cancer may find that this chapter brings your attention to or reminds you of similar emotions you experienced in the past or are experiencing now. This is an important chapter, since unresolved reactions can blunt enjoyment of life, hinder understanding of risk information (Part II), and may even prevent a person from obtaining the breast health care that is right for her.

Part II contains information about breast cancer risks and ways to assess their importance to you. In chapter 2, I show you how different, how relevant, and how clear risk information is when it is presented in formats that are useful to an individual. These formats include the use of a time frame and the reporting of risk in actual or absolute terms instead of as a comparison risk.

You will see that when these "individually useful" formats are used, some of the commonly accepted beliefs about breast cancer risk appear quite different from what you may have heard previously. For example, you will find that breast cancer risks to young women have *not* noticeably increased since the 1970s, that women living in the "high-risk areas" have risks that are not substantially higher than women living in other locations, that the death rate due to breast cancer is decreasing, and that for the growing numbers of women whose breast cancers are found at a small size and have not spread beyond the breast, *the survival to twenty years is over 90%*, usually without chemotherapy!

If you've wondered about what triggers a geneticist's suspicion that a particular family has an increased hereditary risk of cancer, chapter 2 will provide some of the answers. Here I present information about breast cancer risks to women who have a family history of breast cancer, along with an explanation about why two women with identically appearing family histories can have very different risks. The importance of the father's family history in assessing a woman's breast cancer risk is discussed, as is male breast cancer.

In chapter 3, I show you, in a clear step-by-step fashion, how cancer cells arise. You will learn about the amazingly simple changes that can occur in a non-cancer cell to change it into one that is cancerous. Once you understand how cancer cells arise, you, like many of my patients, may find that you are able to think about cancer in a more matter-of-fact fashion. You will also read about the different ways in which hereditary and nonhereditary cancers arise and how this fits in with the tendency of hereditary cancers to occur at younger ages. Chapter 3 includes a straightforward explanation about chromosomes, genes, and gene changes (mutations) and their role in the development of a cancer cell. This is a fascinating story that will set the stage for genetic testing, which I discuss in chapter 4.

In chapter 4 you will read about cancer risks to women who have inherited a mutation (genetic change) in either of two genes—BRCA1 (Breast Cancer 1) or BRCA2 (Breast Cancer 2)—not just breast cancer risk, but risk of ovarian and other cancers as well. This chapter will provide you with information about the likelihood of finding a BRCA mutation and may help you to decide whether genetic testing might be useful for you and/or your family. You will also find information about the risk of cancer to a woman's second breast. In this chapter I describe the types of cancers that may be found in families that have mutations in some of the *non-BRCA genes* for which genetic testing is also available.

Chapter 5 looks at the different types of benign breast disease (fibrocystic breast disease). It explains why most women who have benign breast disease are not at increased risk of breast cancer, which women do have an increased risk, and what the magnitude of this risk actually is. From this discussion you will understand why an accurate assessment of the type of benign breast disease you may have plays such an important role. Chapter 8 shows ways to help you obtain it.

Precancer, cancer—what's in a name? Lots, as chapter 5 explains. Here I discuss two conditions, ductal carcinoma in situ and lobular carcinoma in situ, showing how they differ from each other and from invasive cancer. You will learn why ductal carcinoma in situ incidence has dramatically increased in the last ten years; the importance of learning its type and extent before making a treatment decision; and ways to understand the often contradictory information about prognosis and treatments for the in situ cancers, including the use of radiation therapy for ductal carcinoma in situ. Here I put in context the "increased risk" of cancer to the second breast when a woman has been diagnosed with lobular carcinoma in situ. With this information, you will be better prepared to participate meaningfully in the decision-making process following a diagnosis of an in situ "carcinoma."

Everyone has questions about hormone replacement therapy (HRT). Often you read that "the jury is still out" regarding hormone use and breast cancer risk. But is it? In chapter 6 you will be surprised to see how much we *do know*—certainly enough for you to make an informed decision about HRT use with regard to breast cancer risk and to feel comfortable about it. In chapter 6, I summarize the substantial amount of information we now have about *lack of a relevant increase* in breast cancer risk to women who use HRT at menopause. Here you will also learn how to assess the likelihood that a particular study's results can provide you with reliable information. These tools can help you to avoid being taken in by sensationally reported risks about any topic. For those of you who are tired of reading conflicting information about hormones, this chapter will be an eye-opener.

Many people these days are concerned about the effects of diet and alcohol consumption on their breast cancer risk. In chapter 7 you will find a discussion about what is and is not known about these factors and breast cancer risks—and why. This chapter also examines breast cancer risk to women who use birth control pills. The effects of various aspects of a woman's reproductive history, such as her age at the time of her first period, are reviewed. You will see here that early age at first period, late age at menopause, and childlessness actually play a very minor role in an individual woman's breast cancer risk. Finally, I discuss risk to those who have two risk factors, such as women who have not given birth to a child and who also have a strong family history of cancer.

Part III focuses on ways to use the information you have obtained in Part II. In chapter 8 you will find tips about how to better navigate the medical system when you have a breast concern, including the types of specialists to consult and ways to pose questions that will increase your chances of receiving unbiased, straightforward answers from them. You will also learn about second opinions and their usefulness in helping you to obtain the breast health care and follow-up that you want.

The increasingly important areas of Cancer Risk Assessment and genetic testing are covered in chapter 9. Here you will learn what to look for in a Cancer Risk Assessment service, pitfalls in some common methods of risk assessment, and the role of genetic testing in the Cancer Risk Assessment process. This chapter presents examples of the types of emotions that can arise when individuals receive genetic testing results and some of the issues involved in deciding to have genetic testing.

Chapter 10 contains information to help you make informed decisions about your breast health care. I discuss the two most frequently used methods to detect breast cancer—mammography and physical breast examinations. I also present information for you to consider in making decisions about the so-called preventive measures: prophylactic mastectomy, prophylactic oophorectomy, and the drugs tamoxifen and raloxifene. Here again, the difference between what you have heard and the actual study results may surprise you.

Chapter 11 describes approaches that have helped my patients to live with the uncertainty that is present in all our lives, regardless of breast cancer risk. Here I offer three steps to help you live with this uncertainty, along with several simple but effective exercises. These exercises have helped many of my patients to live more comfortably and peacefully with their breast cancer risks, whatever they are. I present them here in the hope that one or more may help you, too.

The chapters in *Assess Your True Risk of Breast Cancer* contain numerous examples from my twenty-year Cancer Risk Assessment practice in which I have assessed cancer risk and have helped people to understand their risks, to make use of risk information, and to live more comfortably with risk. I think you will find that the figures, tables, risk assessment techniques, and individual stories presented throughout the book will also help you to deepen your ability to assess and evaluate risk and will allow you to feel more assured that you can do so without having to rely on someone else's judgment. In addition, you will achieve greater clarity about the usefulness of genetic testing to you and your family. It is my deep hope that this book will enable you to obtain a clearer understanding of breast cancer risks and that from this understanding you will develop an increased sense of personal power that will lead to a greater sense of security as you make the decisions that are right for you.

Part I

THE
HUMAN
PART

Those Emotions We
Know So Well—Or Do We?

When I got up this morning and saw the news about breast cancer risk, I said, "Oh, no!" My stomach has been in a knot all day.

   —Sabrina, whose sister and mother had breast cancer

Breast cancer is a disease that concerns most modern women. So it should be no surprise that when someone close—her mother, sister, aunt, grandmother, friend, or coworker—is diagnosed with breast cancer, a woman often experiences powerful and long-lasting emotions. As you might expect, a woman's feelings are likely to be stronger when someone she knows well is diagnosed with breast cancer. In this case she will generally learn more details, and be more aware of treatments and ongoing consequences than when a casual acquaintance is diagnosed. Those who are young when a relative is diagnosed may find that their previously stable and secure world is shaken, at least temporarily. A woman whose mother is diagnosed with breast cancer may develop particular sensitivities to the disease and her own chances of having similar experiences, sensitivities that can last for years.

You may think that all of this goes without saying. However, I frequently see women who have had tremendously difficult experiences with a dear one's breast cancer and who still truly believe that their fear of cancer is unreasonably deep, that their fear or concern has arisen from some fault or weakness of their own, and that their feelings are unique or highly unusual. These are apologetic people who reluctantly express their concern with a sigh, a tear, or say with an embarrassed laugh that they are "cancerphobic." When I learn about their experiences, I find that they are *not* cancerphobic at all. Their feelings about cancer are not at all unreasonable, overly strong, or irrational. Instead, they are usually healthy, normal people responding in a most reasonable and understandable way to a powerful formative life experience with a loved one's breast cancer. And, far from being alone in their concern, it is shared by many other women with similar experiences.

Of course, women's experiences with their relatives' cancers differ. Some who were initially quite shaken found that their lives soon returned to "almost normal." For others, the cancer diagnosis in a relative became a turning point in their lives. Whatever these experiences were, most had little or no help in achieving an understanding or assessment of their feelings at the time or those that arose or lingered in the following years. The consequences of this lack of exploration and integration can be profound.

For example, Gloria, a woman in her late forties, whose mother was diagnosed when she was in college, told me:

> I was traveling back and forth, but it was hard for my family to pay my airfare. I couldn't stand to stay home and watch her in pain. So I often stayed away or left early. Mother hated for me to be there and wanted me to be there at the same time. Our family situation deteriorated. All of the children married people we wouldn't have otherwise. We all got away from home in the only acceptable way.

Even though Gloria realized that the course of her life and her siblings' lives was drastically changed as a result of her mother's illness, she was surprised to learn that her concerns about cancer risk were perfectly normal and that they are shared by many other women whose mothers also had breast cancer. Until her visit with me, she had hardly spoken to anyone about her mother's diagnosis and illness. Many of the women I see, like Gloria, had also not spoken to others about their experiences or the emotions arising from them. Many feel different from and even isolated from others, and blame themselves for these feelings as well. If this is your situation, I want you to be aware that whatever your experiences with breast cancer or other potentially serious illness, your feelings about them may well influence how you respond to your chances of developing breast cancer and to your breast health care.

We now have classes for pregnant women, for women who want to learn how to scuba dive, invest in real estate or play golf, but usually not for women (or girls, boys, or men) who have a friend or relative diagnosed with breast cancer. Without access to information about what is normal in such circumstances, without help in coping with their often strong emotions, without an opportunity to reflect on and adapt to the great changes in family functioning that often follow a breast cancer diagnosis, it is no wonder that many women struggle for years to understand and live at peace with their emotions and memories.

If you also have not had an opportunity to explore the thoughts and emotions that arose from your experiences with cancer, you may find that they cast a shadow over your enjoyment of life and may even prevent you from making appropriate health care decisions. You may well find, as many others have, that when these sometimes frightening and unpleasant past experiences are brought forward and examined, you achieve an increased sense of peace and relief. The very process of examination often transforms the experience.

Even if you are someone who thinks there is no reason to "dig up the past," or to "live through all that again," or that you want to "leave well enough alone," I hope you will read on in this chapter about others' experiences with cancer. As you do, I encourage you to think about and write down ways in which *you* have been influenced by your past experiences with breast cancer. Briefly consider if any of these reactions might hinder you from obtaining and using breast cancer risk information or acting on it to set up an effective breast health program. Write down whatever comes up for you. You may want to refer to this list as you read the chapters in Part III.

Beliefs about Cancer's Causes

Most of us have beliefs about the causes of breast cancer. Some fit with current scientific findings and some don't. Whatever your beliefs may be, unless you are aware of them, they may prevent you from hearing or understanding information that differs from them—information that could be useful to you. You might take a minute now to write down some of your beliefs about the causes of cancer and the likely outcome if you should be diagnosed with breast cancer. You will want to compare your beliefs with the information presented in chapter 2 and elsewhere in this book.

Beliefs differ widely. You may believe that since you look like your mother and your sister does not, you probably inherited more of your mother's genes than your sister did and so are more likely to be diagnosed with breast cancer than your sister. Or you might believe that your risk is high, no matter what a risk assessment shows, since "bad things always happen to me."

One way to focus on your beliefs is to ask yourself when and how you came to hold them. You may remember that when your relative was diagnosed with breast cancer a doctor told you, "It's not a matter of *whether* you will get breast cancer but *when*." These are powerful words from an authority figure. Hearing them, you may have assumed (incorrectly, I might add) that you were doomed.

Often, when a person has a chance to discuss her childhood, teenage, young adult, or even mature adult experiences with a friend's or relative's breast cancer, she learns that her beliefs and the information she obtained have remained frozen since that time. Was this your experience? If so, know that it is one that is shared by many. And, like many, you will probably find that once the beliefs and information are explored from today's adult perspective, they can "thaw out," enabling you to see and feel them in a new and less threatening way. With this thaw, any feeling of being "doomed" or "different from others" may well diminish or even disappear.

Anxiety, Worry, Fear

⚭ Some women tell me that when they try to listen to information about breast cancer risk, they hear a roaring in their ears, their "brain turns to cotton candy," or they quickly forget what they have heard. Many say apologetically, "I know I've asked you this before, but I just can't seem to remember what you said." For these people, an inability to understand and retain information is due to a thoroughly understandable anxiety about what they might hear. Those who are afraid that I might tell them they have a "high risk," or that I might give them "bad news" or "scary information" often tune out whatever I say. Unfortunately, they then can't hear useful or reassuring news, either. You might want to make a note of times that you had difficulty hearing information and try to identify what kept you from listening.

When you are anxious or worried about your breast cancer risk, try to remember that nothing is as frightening as the unknown. And, even more important for now, nothing you read here can be as scary as what you have already imagined. You are probably reading this book to learn about your risk so you can set up a reasonable, effective plan for your breast care. And this *can* be done! Many women share your fears or concerns. You, like others, have the capacity to stand back a little from these concerns in order to listen and learn. When you do so you may find that the landscape that was present earlier has changed somewhat because of the new information you received.

As I said earlier, women who had a close friend or relative with breast cancer are frequently more concerned about their breast cancer risk than others who have not had this experience. If, as a child or teenager you took emotional or physical care of the adults around you, you may worry that if you should be diagnosed with breast cancer you will be a burden to others or that your children will suffer as you did. Or, like Jennifer, your fear may be combined with great sorrow:

> I'm thirty and I still cry every time I think about it. I don't know when I'll ever give that up. Not knowing your mother is a strange thing because you don't get an impression of the person you might become. It makes me afraid, of course, that I'm going to die of breast cancer. When I don't express myself, when I'm unhappy I worry most, 'cause I feel I'm acting like my mother and therefore I'm going to die.

Even if your friend or relative survived breast cancer you may be anxious about your quality of life should you develop breast cancer. Fran feared a diagnosis of breast cancer from the time of her aunt's diagnosis: "Emotionally, I don't think my aunt's ever gotten over it. She's lived like the cancer was going to recur and I know she's never felt the same. She's never adjusted to her breast being gone." Darlene, whose mother was diagnosed with breast cancer when she was a child, and is alive and well many years later, had a similar response: "I saw that breast cancer changes and limits your life. And if you like your life the way it is now, you don't want it to be changed or limited."

Jennifer, Fran, and Darlene's reactions are not unusual. You may be helped, as they were, by becoming aware of the many advances that have occurred and are continuing to occur in the area of early breast cancer detection and breast cancer treatment. (I'll discuss improved survival rates in chapter 2.) You may already be aware that treatment has improved—you may know that far fewer mastectomies are done now than in the past, for example, and that when they are performed now far less tissue is removed—but on an emotional level you may not realize that if you were to be diagnosed with breast cancer, your experience would be far different from that of your friend or relative who was diagnosed some years ago. Obtaining information about improvements in techniques and consciously applying these improvements to any situation you might encounter may go far toward reducing your anxiety.

Of course, people differ, so it may be useful to think about your particular assumptions. In some cases a woman can be so used to living with her concern, or even fear, that she no longer realizes she has it. The concern or worry becomes as comfortable (and uncomfortable) as a worn-out, broken-down shoe. Sondra, a 38-year-old woman whose mother and sister were diagnosed with breast cancer, didn't realize how concerned she was. She wasn't able to tell me about her concerns directly, and so said, "I think people are afraid, so afraid. They don't know what will happen. They don't know if it will do any good or not to run from breast cancer." Sondra was talking about her own fear and her own lack of concrete information. She had previously been too afraid to listen carefully to details or to have careful breast care. Once she learned what she could do to protect herself and started a more rigorous follow-up program, she found that some of the tension in her life, tension brought about in part by her breast cancer fears, was greatly reduced.

Fear about breast cancer can spread into all aspects of a woman's life. Sally, who had several friends with breast cancer, said, "When I get sick with anything, I worry about breast cancer." Denise, a 52-year-old woman with a family history of breast cancer, confided, "It's always in the back of your mind. You get busy and you forget it, but it's always there when you get right down to it." As these comments suggest, once a person has a deep concern about cancer, worrying can become a habit. Some women, like Deanna, endure cycles of worry:

> I've never ever gotten over being scared. My sister and I have never really talked about it in depth. During the whole time Mom was sick we could never talk about it. We could never even bring it up. It would be too scary for us together. When it comes up I usually cry a lot and then it dissipates. And then it's over. But it repeats itself a lot.

Harriet, a very perceptive woman in her late thirties, noticed that she suffered from recurrent anxiety. When she looked at this more closely she realized:

> Often when I'm getting worried about my breasts, it's a signal to me that something else is going on and that the something else isn't getting taken care of. Whenever I pay attention to *that* pressure and resolve it, that helps to take care of my breast cancer fear.

Fear, worries, and anxieties such as these can have a major influence on the quality of your life and on your family's sense of well-being. When you become impatient with any remaining fear or anxiety, it might help you to consider that fear can have a positive effect, too—an aspect that is often not appreciated. For example, fear can help to remind you that something needs to be done even when you try to avoid it or not think about it. Fear can help you to notice that a situation is dangerous and requires your attention. Until you are clear about what needs to be done and do it, fear can be uncomfortable. The discomfort, seen in this light, is actually a friend and a helper. The point is to channel this fear, discomfort, or unease into useful action and not be incapacitated by it or live with it for long periods of time. The chapters in Part III are designed to help you make informed health care decisions about your breasts, work effectively with the health care system, and explore approaches and exercises that can help you live more comfortably with uncomfortable emotions.

Guilt

༒ Few, if any of us, can look back on our lives without experiencing some sense of guilt. If a friend or relative had breast cancer you may think, "If only I had done something to help" or "If only I had helped more." Many, many women have expressed these sentiments to me over the years, even those who did a tremendous amount for a loved one. Because these women had no opportunity to speak about and explore their experiences in a meaningful manner, many carried feelings of guilt with them for years. Once they had a chance to talk about and think through their past, no matter how difficult, most were amazed to realize that in previous years, no matter what they did or didn't do, they were actually doing the best they could under extremely difficult circumstances.

If you were a child, teenager, or young adult when your mother was diagnosed with breast cancer you, too, may feel guilty, even years later, if you believe that you didn't help your mother enough when she was ill or weren't sympathetic about her fear and pain. Polly remembered:

> I was feeling real impatient and angry with her for being so ill and not being able to go out with us any more. She needed so much help! And I felt so angry all the time so I didn't give her all the help she needed.

Anne, who was also a teenager when her mother was diagnosed with breast cancer, had a similar reaction:

> I was just feeling impatient. I didn't even feel sorry for her. I was feeling sorry for myself and I was running away a lot. I spent most of my time going out with friends. It was terrible of me.

Alexandra, who was a young adult when her mother found a breast lump, didn't take it at all seriously or talk to her mother about its significance. She reported:

> When I got to the hospital my mother already had the mastectomy. That was something I never expected, so I wasn't there to give her the support she needed.

For each of these women, guilt had accumulated over decades.

When you have a chance to look at your past experiences from a more mature perspective, you will probably see that when you were younger your ability to help was far more limited than you felt it to be at the time. Those of you who were teenagers or young adults when your mother had breast cancer and who are adults now can appreciate how normal it is for individuals of that age to want to establish their independence. Your mother's illness occurred at a time when normal developmental processes were leading you to increasingly separate yourself from her. Naturally you struggled to maintain your newfound sense of a separate self and did not want to be concerned with your mother's health. You were then a girl or young woman who was involved in the normal separation process that comes with growing up.

Once you have an opportunity to talk about and review your past, you are likely to have a different perspective of your behaviors then *and* your feelings now. This review of events, even events that were quite painful, can be like creating order in a room with jumbled furniture. Even if no new furniture is added to the room, the changed arrangement (in this case a changed perspective) creates a very different feeling. With understanding and clarity comes a sense of forgiveness for all involved, including yourself, and a lessening of any guilt feelings. As Eileen said when she understood her situation as a teenager:

> To think I've been carrying that guilt around all these years. I felt so grown up then and so responsible, but now I see that I was just a kid. What could I have known then?

Guilt is, of course, a most unpleasant feeling. It can be such a heavy burden that it greatly diminishes a person's quality of life. From a sense of guilt, a woman may even come unconsciously to believe that her past action (or inaction) means that she is not worthy of information, of good medical care, or even of an effective breast health plan. In these cases, unresolved feelings of guilt that arise from feeling, for example, that she has emotionally betrayed a friend or relative, may put a woman's very life at risk. That is an important reason to resolve these issues and move on with your life.

You may be surprised to realize that guilt feelings, even those that are quite painful, can at times serve a useful purpose. You may find, for instance, that guilt feelings helped you to feel more in control of a situation in which you actually had very little power or influence. By feeling guilty for not doing more or for not making the situation better, you may have been able to avoid acknowledging that you were powerless to "fix" it or to make a terrible situation any better. In this way, a feeling of guilt for not doing "enough" may have helped to protect you from fear and may even have prevented you from being emotionally overwhelmed by the situation. It is unresolved guilt, guilt that goes on for years, that can be particularly harmful. By recognizing that guilt may have served a purpose at one time, you can often move beyond these feelings to an increased sense of ease. Of course, your situation may be different. Here I offer examples of what has been so for the women I have seen for Cancer Risk Assessment.

Beliefs about Survival

⅋ Some women whose mothers had breast cancer feel so strongly that they will follow a similar path that they may say things like "I can feel in my bones that I'll get breast cancer." Or "I know that some day I'll have breast cancer, just like my mother." Even a woman who consciously tries to be different from her mother may find that in sometimes incredibly subtle ways she is reacting as her mother would. If your mother died of breast cancer, you may come to assume, as many women do, that you will also. Some, like Eliza, remember having these concerns from the time they were children:

> When I was a child I remember thinking something like, well, this means that I will have to die of breast cancer. I was very clear with myself about that. But I told myself that it wouldn't be for a long time. And I think I still have a feeling that this is my fate, just like when I was a kid.

Women who believe that they are destined to develop or die of breast cancer sometimes shape their lives around this expectation. One woman told me she decided to marry a "kind but boring" man who would take good care of her "when" she had breast cancer. She was in her seventies when I saw her, still married and somewhat mystified about why she had *never* developed breast cancer! Another woman said that ever since her mother's breast cancer diagnosis, she expected to be told she had breast cancer each year at her annual exam. Still another, when she learned that she had not inherited the mutation that her mother and grandmother carried, wondered what she would now do with her life. She, like many women, had structured her life and sense of self around the certainty of a breast cancer diagnosis, and so no longer knew who she was or what to do when she learned that it was unlikely she would ever have breast cancer. These women suffer from what I call an "Unlived Life Syndrome" or a "Less than Fully Lived Life Syndrome"—until they sort through the issues.

Some women's experiences have left them with a feeling of helplessness or doom whenever they think about breast cancer. Stella, whose mother and sister were diagnosed with breast cancer, acknowledged, "You feel kind of helpless. You sit there and wait for it to come and there's nothing you can do. I don't like that feeling!" Erica, who felt she resembled her mother a great deal, said, "I've always felt that I probably will have breast cancer. It's weird. I'm not *wishing* it on myself, but it's always a feeling I've had." For some, the reactions are particularly intense. Gerta told me:

> When I found my lump I ran through the alternatives: dying, leaving my husband so I wouldn't put him through hell, biopsy, and so forth. I alternated between feeling that I've had a good life and feeling it's unjust.

Erica and Gerta were aware that their mothers' experiences with breast cancer had shaped their lives and outlook, so they could begin to examine whether their beliefs about risk that were derived from the past actually matched the current reality. Unfortunately, many women whose mothers had breast cancer are unaware that they are carrying an assumption of doom. Such a built-in, yet unconscious, assumption can have far-reaching, negative consequences. A recognition of these assumptions can greatly improve a woman's quality of life.

My experiences with Karen provide a good illustration of some of the changes that can occur when unconscious, negative assumptions about breast cancer are brought into conscious awareness. Karen was a lovely young mother of two little boys. She came to her first visit with her husband, Greg. They were an attractive couple, and obviously cared a great deal for each other. Still, Greg looked grim as he recounted his wife's depression, lack of energy, and inability to enjoy life. "I just don't understand it," he said. "We have each other, we have wonderful children, and she still finds it hard to get out of bed."

Karen began to cry at that point. She said she felt terribly guilty about her depression, reminded herself every day about how lucky she was, but still couldn't seem to enjoy her life. "I feel as if I am living in a heavy cloud," she said. "I am tired all the time and just can't seem to get moving." When I asked Karen about her family history, I learned that her mother was diagnosed with breast cancer shortly after the birth of Karen's younger sister and died four years later, when Karen was six. In the course of our meetings, it became clear that Karen had made an assumption that she would follow in her mother's footsteps and soon die of breast cancer now that her second child was born, just as her mother had.

As Karen began to focus on some of her previously unrecognized assumptions, she began to regain hope and with it energy. The change in her outlook occurred slowly and steadily over several months. Work with a psychotherapist was very helpful to her. Before she could regain hope, she needed to be aware of assumptions she had made about the certainty that she would soon die of breast cancer.

Some women whose mothers died of breast cancer, particularly those who were teenagers or young adults at the time, feel that the loss of their mother has profoundly affected their relationships with others. For example, Lisa told me:

> I still think I have problems getting really close to somebody. I have difficulty trusting people. It's really childish, but I carry this feeling that if you really love something, it's going to die. That's the way I *feel*. Intellectually I know that's not true. But I've had to really work at having a close personal relationship with anybody.

If this is the case for you, it's important to realize that you are not alone in this feeling. I have seen many women who share it. And I have seen many of these women learn how to form and maintain close relationships with others. There are a variety of ways to do this, some of which are described in chapter 11. The first—and most important—step, however, is recognition.

When people feel trapped or isolated, as many women do when their friend or relative has had breast cancer, they may give up and fail to take even the simple steps that could help to protect them. Studies show that individuals who believe they have little control over their health feel less well, have more illness, and are less likely to seek preventive care than those who feel they have more control.[1] If you feel trapped or isolated it is important for you to move beyond this feeling to set up an effective breast health program. As the results of these studies suggest, the benefits will go far beyond better breast health care, and are likely to lead to an increased sense of well-being.

Uncertainty about Appropriate Care

Unwarranted trust, mistrust, or uncertainty about whether to trust health care providers can be bad for your health. These reactions can arise from past painful experiences with the medical profession—your own or those of someone you care for. Helen, who works in the medical field, was negatively influenced by the first doctor her favorite aunt saw:

> So this is what her doctor tells her—"You've got a cancer spread and there's nothing I can do. You might as well live it up in the time you have left." I said, "That's ridiculous! There's all sorts of other tests they can give her before he tells her that." Then when we went to the other doctor and he did more tests, they couldn't find a thing. Her cancer *hadn't* spread.

Even though Helen was able to help her aunt find good medical care, that experience shaped her subsequent approach to doctors. When she meets a new doctor, she says her attitude now is, "Prove to me you are not incompetent." Because Helen is aware that she has these feelings she takes them into account and is careful not to be hasty in judging a new doctor.

Melissa told me that she has difficulty believing what doctors say. She was profoundly affected by the way doctors treated her mother: "My mother's doctors always acted as if she was this silly woman who was always complaining. And she was really sick!" It's no wonder that Melissa now finds herself wondering if she can believe a doctor who says she has no medical problems.

If your experiences have led you to develop a sense of mistrust or unease about doctors or nurses as a group, it's important to remember that there are many wonderful and dedicated health professionals who can help you a great deal and who will take your concerns seriously. It is important to be watchful, while giving yourself time to get acquainted before you make a judgment. New acquaintances are rarely as comfortable as those we know better.

You might think that women who mistrust physicians would see them infrequently. This is often not the case, however. The lack of trust, as well as concerns due to past experiences with cancer, can lead a person to feel uneasy about her health. This, in turn, may result in an increased use of a physician's time, as Juliet explained:

> I don't trust doctors and I have been afraid of them since my mother was sick. I've always been afraid that they will find something really wrong. And I still go a lot—if I have a cold, a sore throat, or something, I just go all the time, which is absurd. I understand real hypochondriacs don't ever go to the doctor, so maybe this means I'm not a true hypochondriac. But all my friends make jokes about how often I go to the doctor. Because I'm so afraid.

Finding a doctor or nurse you can trust and with whom you feel comfortable will help to ensure that you receive good follow-up care and will also help to release you from unwarranted anxiety. Marcy searched before finding the doctor who was right for her:

> The main thing I've done has been to seek out someone who would say, "In my best judgment, you're OK," and I've cast about a bit for that. That's the process I've gone through until I've felt that I'd done my best to find the people I felt would give

me the best chance, who did the most, and who had the most experiences that would be available to me. Once I had done that, then I felt more comfortable than I had ever been before.

I encourage you to do the same. In chapter 8, I'll discuss ways to set up effective breast health care and tell you about ways to evaluate the care you are given.

You may be convinced that you need a useful breast health program, but are uncertain about how to proceed. You, like Amy, may find yourself wondering if you are worrying too much about breast cancer risk or not doing enough:

> You always have this slight anxiety about everything that happens in your body. You're always asking yourself, "Am I being neurotic about this or should I let it go?"

If you believe your breast cancer risk is high, you may find it particularly difficult to feel sure you *are* doing enough. Emily, who has a strong family history of breast cancer, described her dilemma this way:

> There's no magic standard that says if you do this you've done it. The publicity says to examine your own breasts once a month and you're OK. But I'm not sure of that. I flail about a bit and I end up getting a lot of doctor breast exams. If you feel at high risk, it's very difficult to feel like you're doing enough.

Though Emily is right—there *is* no magic standard—guidelines are available to help a woman who feels she is at high risk to identify a high-quality breast health follow-up program. This is discussed in Part III.

Over the years I have found that anxiety is reduced when people have accurate, understandable information and know how to apply it to keep themselves safe. So, read on! Much of the rest of this book is designed to help you do just that.

Part II

JUST
THE FACTS,
MA'AM

TWO

❧❧

Age, Family History, and High-Risk Areas: Decoding the Statistics

How can you ever find out what is true short of becoming a mathematician yourself? The answer is: you don't have to. You merely need the confidence to ask the questions that were probably on your mind anyway. Such as: how do you know? Based on what evidence? Compared to what else?

—K. C. Cole, *The Universe and the Teacup: The Mathematics of Truth and Beauty*[1]

If you are like many of the women I counsel, you may wonder why, with all you have read and heard about breast cancer risk, you are still not clear about many points. With all the studies that have been done, you may ask, why is there still so much conflicting information? Perhaps you feel overwhelmed or confused by news reports and wonder how it can even be possible to make sense of the different breast cancer risks. After all, we know numbers can be manipulated. How can you realistically distinguish between a risk that is important to you and one that is not?

I think you will find that the information in this chapter will give you a context within which to evaluate the usefulness of risks and help you to feel more confident about your ability to do so with ease. As the quotation at the beginning of this chapter points out, much of making sense depends on common sense.

In this chapter I'll be discussing some of the basics about how to assess and interpret breast cancer risks, including risk to the average woman. I'll take a look at the so-called high-risk areas and the risk to women who have a close relative with breast cancer. My patients tell me again and again that these approaches help them to understand risks and to apply them to their lives with a sense of assurance. Read on and you'll see that you can, too!

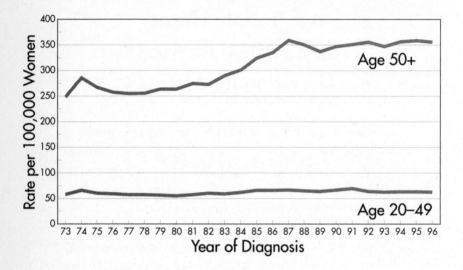

Figure 1. Women's Invasive Breast Cancer Incidence 1973–1996
Source: Adapted from Ries et al., 1999.[2]

Is the Risk Increasing?

◈ Many people ask me why the rate of breast cancer keeps going up and up, especially among younger women. But is it? If you look at figure 1, the National Cancer Institute's breast cancer data for a number of communities across the country from 1973 to 1996 (the last year for which data are available), you will see two lines. The top line represents the number of breast cancer cases per 100,000 women diagnosed with breast cancer at age 50 and older. As you can see, the rate was fairly steady from 1991 to 1995. Remember that these are the rates per 100,000 women, so the slight rise in 1987 and the dip in 1989 represent fewer than 25 women *out of 100,000*. These are very minor changes that can seem larger or more important than they are unless you pay close attention to the actual numbers that are and are not affected.

You can also see in figure 1 that from the late 1970s to the late 1980s the breast cancer rate in older women increased steadily, after which you will notice a leveling off of the rate. Be aware that this rise, which may appear large on the graph, again represents very few women. It is a change from about 250 cases per 100,000 in 1978 to about 360 per 100,000 in 1988, a difference of about 110 women *per 100,000 women.* In percentage this is a change from 0.25% in 1978 to 0.36% in 1988. Can you see how important it is to determine the size of the group in which breast cancers are found?

The increase in breast cancer rate from the late 1970s to late 1980s was probably due to a number of factors, among them:

- Use of better methods to collect and report the numbers of women diagnosed with breast cancer
- Increased probability of finding breast cancers due to:
  - Improvements in the quality of mammography
  - Improvements in training radiologists (the physicians who read mammograms)
  - A growing awareness among women and physicians about the value of early breast cancer detection, leading to a greater frequency of physical breast examinations and breast biopsies, which in turn increase the number of breast cancers that are detected

Many breast cancers that are now found would, in previous years, have been undetected during a woman's entire lifetime. Before a woman's breast cancer would have grown large enough to be detected, she would have died of other causes. In other words, much or all of the increase in women 50 and older in figure 1 appears to be due to improved detection and reporting and not to an increase in the number of breast cancers that occurred.

Now let's take a look at the lower line in figure 1, which represents breast cancers diagnosed in women up to age 50. As you can see, the breast cancer rate—again, the number diagnosed per 100,000—has been fairly steady *and has not increased substantially since the 1970s.* If you take into account most women's greater awareness of breast cancer and the increased use of early detection techniques, the lack of an increase in breast cancer rates in younger women is actually quite surprising.

So, as you can see, the national breast cancer rates in figure 1 simply do not support the perception that breast cancer is a growing epidemic.

Why, then, do we hear so much more about it than ever before? At least part of the answer lies in the growing interest in and awareness of this disease. Until recently many women hid a diagnosis of breast cancer from their children, from their friends, and from the community at large. Now, to a much greater extent, women are more comfortable sharing their experiences with others and receiving support from family, friends, and the community—opportunities that were not available years ago. For example, many women now join support groups after their diagnosis. This increased willingness to discuss breast cancer means that we *hear* about it more often, but it does not mean it is *happening* with the great increase in frequency that most of us have come to believe.

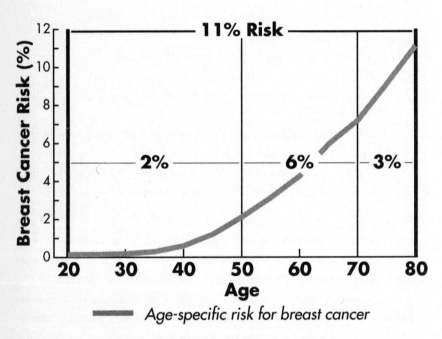

Figure 2. Age and Breast Cancer Risk
Source: Adapted from Ries et al., 1999.

Average Risk: 1 in 8, 1 in 9

One statistic you've probably heard again and again is that the average woman's breast cancer risk is about 1 in 9 or 1 in 8. It is important for you to understand what this risk actually means. A risk of 1 in 9 (which is 11%) represents the average woman's risk *from age 20 to 80*. The 1 in 8 includes a risk to even older ages—to over 100. Take a look at figure 2. As you can see from the heavy dark line, a woman's chance of being diagnosed with breast cancer increases with age. For women 20 to 50, the average risk is just 2%, from 50 to 70 it is 6%, and from 70 to 80 it is 3%. The 11% or 1 in 9 is obtained by adding the risk in each age category, 2% + 6% + 3% = 11%.

When a woman who has the average risk reaches age 50 without a diagnosis of breast cancer, she has passed through 2% of her risk so her risk to age 80 is now 11% minus 2%, which equals 9%. When she reaches 70 without a diagnosis of breast cancer, her risk to age 80 is then 11% − 2% − 6% = 3%. You can see that time must be included with a risk figure if that risk is to be meaningful. Also, a woman's risk can be stated in different ways by using different time frames. For example, the average 50-year-old woman's risk is 6% to age 70, but 9% to age 80.

When I reviewed this material with Gail, a patient of mine, she shook her head, sighed, and said, "Are you saying that two percent of a person's risk can just disappear when she reaches fifty?" I asked Gail to think of it this way: she faced certain risks driving her car to come and see me for her appointment. Once she reached my office safely, only the risk for her return trip remained. In the same way, as she travels through each year without a breast cancer diagnosis, the risk associated with that year is gone. I also pointed out that, in any given year, older women are at higher risk than younger women, but the closer they come to 80, the more their risk *to age 80* diminishes, because they have fewer years ahead of them before age 80 than do younger women.

Carrying this comparison one more step, I suggested that Gail think of a busy street that a woman must cross every year of her life. In a single trip (which here would represent a single year's breast cancer risk) a younger woman, being more agile than an older woman, is less likely to be hit by a car. However, a younger woman also has more trips ahead of her in her lifetime than does an older woman, and so has a higher *lifetime* risk. This example can be applied to breast cancer: there is one risk for any given year based on a woman's age and a higher risk up to age 80 because more years are included. Although 11% is the average woman's risk from age 20 to age 80, this number does not accurately reflect any one woman's risk at any particular time.

I want to emphasize how fundamental it is to the discussion of breast cancer risk—or any other risk—that a measure of time be included. *Risk without a time frame is simply not informative.* Many of us are aware that this is true for speed as well: to say that an object is traveling at 50 miles does not provide useful information. For it to be useful, we need to know whether the speed refers to, say, 50 miles per hour or 50 miles per second. It is the same with breast cancer risk. No one can evaluate the magnitude or importance of a risk without an accompanying time frame. Also, without an understanding that risk gets "used up" over time, you have no useful way to evaluate a risk's significance to you now, in the next five years, and beyond.

As she examined figure 2, Gail asked why women 70 to 80 had a 3% risk, compared to the 6% for women from 50 to 70—"Doesn't a woman's breast cancer risk increase with age?" Yes, I told her, the risk does go up with age. Here again, a careful look at the time frame is critical: the 3% risk covers only 10 years (70 to 80), while the 6% risk covers 20 years (50 to 70). Risk and time must be considered together.

"High-Risk" Areas

 My practice is in the San Francisco Bay Area, which is said to have one of the highest rates of breast cancer in the country. Therefore, many of the women I see are particularly concerned that something in their neighborhood might be contributing to an increased risk of breast cancer.

As you may have heard, higher breast cancer rates tend to be found in higher socioeconomic areas. Some people have speculated that there are environmental or reproductive (see chapter 7) causes for these higher rates. But think about it: the women who live in higher socioeconomic areas are often highly mobile; many did not grow up in these "high-risk" locations, and have been exposed to their so-called high-risk environment often for relatively few years.

What, then, do women from the high-risk areas have in common? Consider these factors: upscale communities tend to have more physicians and more highly educated and health-conscious women who tend to seek prompt treatment for any health problem. Studies clearly show that women from higher socioeconomic groups are more likely to seek mammograms and physical breast examinations and to insist on breast biopsies than women with fewer economic resources. Taken together, these factors lead to a far greater likelihood that breast cancers will be found in women from higher socioeconomic groups—leading to a reporting of "increased risk" in their areas.

I was surprised to learn how little the actual *number* of women with breast cancer differs between the high- and low-rate areas. For example, from 1992 to 1996, the last years for which national figures of this type were available, the San Francisco Bay Area had a breast cancer rate of about 115 *per 100,000 women,* Connecticut had about 117, and the lowest rate was in Utah—about 95 per 100,000.

"Okay," you say, "but if I'm one of those 'additional' women who is diagnosed with breast cancer, it still means *I have it.*" Yes, that's true. No matter how low the risk, no one wants to be diagnosed with breast cancer. That's why it's so important for you to know the risks, to be able to put them in perspective, and to learn what you can do.

Every day you probably make choices to minimize possible dangers in your life, even though you realize you can't eliminate them. You may carefully turn off the stove, lock the house or car doors, look both ways before crossing the street, wear a seat belt, etc. You realize that even with precautions, accidents or illness can occur, but you feel better by having a plan that keeps you as safe as possible. If you wear a seat belt and drive responsibly, you may tend to worry less about being in an accident, even though you know full well that another car could still hit yours.

Many people find that their concerns about a risk are reduced when they know that they are doing all that can be done, and that the measures they take will be useful. It's the same with breast cancer. The point is not to discredit the effects of the environment on breast cancer risk. Instead, I want you to realize that environmental factors are unlikely to account for the differences in breast cancer rates found in higher and lower socioeconomic areas of the country.

Early Detection and Breast Cancer Survival

So far in this chapter I've shown you that some of the more commonly held beliefs about breast cancer risk are quite different from the actual facts. But what if a woman is diagnosed with breast cancer? Here you may find that the survival rates are far more hopeful than you had realized. In fact, when a breast cancer is found before it reaches a little less than half an inch in size, *it is almost never life threatening.*

Size

When I first started my practice, over twenty years ago, the average breast cancer was larger than 2 centimeters (cm) in size when it was discovered. Figure 3 shows the actual sizes of different breast lumps, using both centimeters and inches. You can see that a 2 cm lump is about the size of a penny. These days, in many communities where women have yearly mammograms and at least yearly physical breast examinations, breast cancers tend to be found in the 1.5 cm or smaller range—less than the size of a dime. In fact, many breast cancers can be felt before they even reach 1 cm—a little less than half an inch. Mammograms can detect breast cancers that are still smaller.

The wonderful fact is, breast cancers that measure 1 cm or less are unlikely to recur, whether they are treated with surgical removal of the tumor (lumpectomy) followed by radiation treatment or with removal of the entire breast (mastectomy). And with breast cancers this small, chemotherapy and tamoxifen treatments are usually not needed.

Let's take a look at some of the studies of women whose breast cancers were found at a small size. In one, where the breast cancers measured up to 1 cm when they were found, the *sixteen-year* survival from breast cancer was about 90%.[3] In other studies, similar excellent survivals are found. For example, in one study of women whose breast cancers were 1 cm or

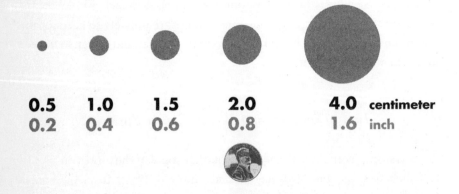

Figure 3. Breast Cancers of Different Sizes

less in size at the time they were found, the breast cancer survival rate all the way up to twenty years was 83%.[4]

You might wonder how easy it is to find breast cancers when they are small. My physician and nurse colleagues tell me that in many women's breasts they have felt breast cancers that were as small as 0.3 cm. Of course, mammography can pick up breast cancers even smaller than that. Nationally, from 1983 to 1996, each year a higher and higher proportion of breast cancers has been found at smaller, more curable sizes.

Cancer in Lymph Nodes

One reason that a breast cancer's size at detection is so important is that the smaller the breast cancer, the more likely it is that cancer is present only in the breast. With small breast cancers there is little chance that cancer cells have traveled to the lymph nodes under the arm or to other parts of the body. Women with small breast cancers who have no cancer cells in the lymph nodes have even better survival rates than women with small breast cancers as a group. For example, in one study women whose breast cancers measured less than 1 cm and whose lymph nodes were free of tumor had a 99% *survival* up to twelve years.[5] Other studies report similar excellent survival rates. In another recent study that followed women with these small breast cancers, women whose lymph nodes were free of cancer had a 92% breast cancer survival up to twenty years.[6]

These excellent survival figures surprise many people. I am often asked if the results of studies such as these are a fluke. I am pleased to report that there are now a number of studies with similar findings.

You can see that when breast cancers are found at small sizes few women die of this disease. In general, the smaller a woman's breast cancer, the less likely that her lymph nodes will have cancer cells in them and the better her prognosis will be. I don't want to mislead you here: a woman can be diagnosed with a small breast cancer and still have cancer in the lymph nodes. Usually, however, when a breast cancer is small, the lymph nodes will be free of cancer cells. (As discussed in chapter 5, new methods can detect very small numbers of cancer cells in the lymph nodes, but cells found using these newer methods appear to lack the ability to cause disease elsewhere since they are found in groups of women who do not develop metastatic disease.) For that matter, some women who have large breast cancers, with cancer found in many nodes, remain well and healthy for years. There are, as you can see, no absolutes, but the generalizations do hold for most women.

Declining Death Rates

As you just read, women whose breast cancers are found at small sizes rarely have cancer recur and almost never die of breast cancer. In recent years, increasing numbers of breast cancers have been found at smaller sizes due to the improvements in early detection techniques discussed previously. As women's breast cancers decreased in size, breast cancer rates started to drop. Since the late 1980s, the breast cancer death rate has fallen and is likely to continue to decrease as more and more breast cancers are found at smaller sizes.

When a Relative Has Breast Cancer

> I just feel that my daughters are programmed to get breast cancer. I've had it and my sister died of it. I worry all the time about my girls. What a terrible legacy I've given them.
> —Joyce, 57, with two daughters in their thirties

Like Joyce, many of the women I see believe that almost all cancers are hereditary. They assume that if a woman has breast cancer, her daughter will almost certainly also be affected. Their daughters share this concern. I regularly hear sentiments such as the following from them:

- "To me, it's not a question of whether I'll get it, but when."
- "I've always known it would happen to me one day, too."
- "I feel like a walking time bomb."
- "Since I look more like my mother than my sister does, I know I'm the one who will get it."

Many of the women I see are surprised to discover that *about 85% of all breast cancers are not due to strong hereditary factors.* About 10% of all breast cancers occur in a family more frequently than would be expected by chance, but no strong hereditary factor appears to be present. Only about 5%, and perhaps up to 8 or 10%, of all breast cancers are thought to be due to strong hereditary factors. (The origin of strong hereditary cancers is described in chapter 3.)

If you have a family history of breast cancer, you will probably be greatly relieved and reassured to learn about the effectiveness of early detection techniques and the excellent survival rates women have when their breast cancers are diagnosed at small sizes. You may be further surprised to learn that most women who have a mother or sister with breast cancer never develop this disease. In fact, most women who have *both* a mother and sister with breast cancer *do not* develop breast cancer!

When I say that most women who have a close affected relative will not get breast cancer, individuals sometimes assume that they haven't heard me correctly or that I have misspoken. Once, two sisters called me to say that they had read this statement in a brochure describing my Cancer Risk Assessment practice and wanted to let me know that I had made a mistake. After all, they told me, they had often heard that if a woman has a mother or sister with breast cancer, her risk is two or three times greater than that of a woman who has no close affected relative.

I assured these young women that I had not made a mistake and invited them to come and see me to learn why the statement they heard and what I had written were both correct—as far as they went. That is, women who have a mother or sister with breast cancer *do* have a breast cancer risk that is two or three times higher than that of women without such a family history *and still* most women who have a close relative with breast cancer will never be diagnosed with this disease.

Comparison Risks

When I met with the two sisters, I learned, as I suspected, that their confusion arose because they didn't realize that:

- Risks presented as comparisons can be misleading.
- The effects of a mixed group (heterogeneity) need to be taken into account. A study's result applies to the group as a whole, while subgroups within it may have different risks.

First, I discussed comparison risks. I advised them to be wary of risks that are presented as, say, a twofold increase in risk or a 40% decrease in risk. When risks are presented this way you are generally not told two times higher than *what* or 40% less than *what*. The "what" is called the baseline risk. If the baseline group (for example, women whose mother or a sister does not have breast cancer) has a risk of 5% over the next 20 years, a twofold increase in risk would mean a risk of 10% over 20 years (5% × 2 = 10%). But if the baseline group has a risk of 0.5%, a twofold increase in risk would amount to only 1% in this same time (0.5% × 2 = 1%). You can see that unless you know the risk to the baseline group, a comparison risk is not useful, and may even be misleading.

Another way to look at this might be to suppose that you love to eat at interesting restaurants, but you have some difficulty climbing stairs. One night you have a choice: you can either go to a highly acclaimed restaurant located on the top floor of a building that has no elevator or to a snack bar on the ground floor of the building next door. If you learn that the building with the fine restaurant has twice as many flights of stairs as the building with the snack bar, how useful is this information? Obviously, this method of comparison will not help you to make a decision about where to eat. If the smaller building has one flight of stairs, the one that is twice as high has two flights, which you could probably manage. However, if the smaller building has 15 flights, the excellent restaurant is 30 flights up— probably too far for you to climb. To make an informed decision, you need to know how many flights there actually are. The "actually are" figure is sometimes called the absolute risk. In making informed decisions about breast cancer risks, you will find that the absolute or actual risks are more useful than those presented as comparison risks.

When I explained the lack of useful information that is conveyed when comparison risks are used, one of the sisters said she had assumed that she could multiply the twofold increase in risk to women who have an affected mother or sister by the average woman's risk of 11%. I explained that this would not work, since studies don't include women from age 20 all the way up to 80, which is the range covered by the 11% risk.

It is possible to obtain a rough approximation of the absolute risk from a comparison risk, particularly if women's ages in a study span twenty years or less and are about evenly distributed. In these cases, however, the comparison risk would not be multiplied by 11% but by, for example, 2% if women in the study were between the ages of 20 and 50 (see figure 2). In one study, where the comparison risk was 3.5, the absolute risk (the risk in percentages per year without comparing one group's risk to another) was

1% a year. In another study with a comparison risk of 3.4, the absolute risk was 1 in 7,000 a year. The different absolute risks obtained in these two studies were due to very different risks in the baseline group.

Once the sisters understood that comparison risks provide information only about one group's risk in relation to the risk in another group, and that even a large difference in comparison risk between two groups can amount to a small absolute risk, we were ready to proceed. I then told them about the results of two studies of women who had a close relative or relatives with breast cancer. In these studies, the risks were reported as absolute risks, without comparison to another group. In the first study, women whose mother *and* sister were diagnosed with breast cancer were found to have a breast cancer risk of 16% up to age 60.[7] That's right—to age 60 there was an 84% chance that these women would *not* be diagnosed with breast cancer, even though both their mother and sister were affected.

Other studies have shown similar results. One included a group of women whose families had at least two generations of women who were diagnosed with breast cancer. In this study, sisters of affected women had a 20% risk of breast cancer up to age 70.[8] In other words, these women had an 80% chance that they would *not* get breast cancer up to age 70.

Heterogeneity

To understand why most women who have a mother or sister with breast cancer won't be diagnosed with breast cancer, it helps to remember that breast cancer is a fairly common disease. A woman who comes from a large family and who has many long-lived relatives may have several who are diagnosed with breast cancers that are due to nonhereditary factors. Another woman, who has a similar-appearing family history, may have several affected relatives whose breast cancers *are* hereditary. So you can see that in a group of women who have one or more relatives with breast cancer, some of the women will have relatives whose breast cancers are hereditary and some will not.

Women whose relatives' cancers are due to strong hereditary factors may be at greatly increased risk of breast cancer, while those whose relatives' cancers are not due to hereditary factors do not have an increased hereditary risk and may have the average woman's breast cancer risk. Scientists call a mixed group, such as one in which some families have strong hereditary factors and some do not, heterogeneous. No matter how diligently or carefully you study a heterogeneous group *as a group*, you may not obtain accurate information about different types of individuals in it. For example, you won't obtain accurate information about bananas by studying a mixture of apples, oranges, and bananas. Instead, if you want precise information about bananas, you need to be sure that only bananas are included in your study.

Similarly, a group of women having a close relative with breast cancer may include some whose relative's breast cancer is due to strong hereditary factors and some whose relative's breast cancer is not strongly hereditary. Hereditary breast cancers are rare—about 5% to 10% of all breast cancers. Therefore, most of the women with an affected relative will not have an increased hereditary risk.

The sisters I was explaining this to looked a little puzzled, so I suggested that they imagine a cup that is 5% filled with red ink. This cup represents the 5% of women with breast cancer whose disease is due to strong hereditary factors. The close relatives of these women have a greatly increased risk of breast cancer. Next to the cup that is 5% filled with red ink is a cup that is 95% filled with clear water. The second cup with the clear water represents the majority of women with breast cancer—those whose cancer is not due to strong hereditary factors. The close relatives of these women do not have an increased risk of breast cancer due to hereditary factors. If you combine the small amount of red water in one cup with the larger amount of clear water in the other cup, you will obtain a cup completely filled with pink water. When scientists study *all* women who have a mother or sister with breast cancer, they are studying the cup of pink water. The entire group will appear to be at somewhat increased risk—the two- to threefold increase in risk you have heard about—but actually the group is heterogeneous. It is made up of a few who are at greatly increased risk (the red ink) and most whose risk is not increased (the majority, the clear water).

The sisters got it. Once they understood this important concept—and once you understand it—you will be better able to interpret results of studies on other factors: risks to carriers of mutations in the BRCA genes (see chapter 4), risks to women who are diagnosed with benign breast disease or ductal carcinoma in situ (see chapter 5), risks associated with alcohol consumption, with childlessness (see chapter 7), and with other risk factors.

Many people assume that if even a single person in their family has breast cancer, the risks to close relatives must be greatly increased. The concept of heterogeneity can help them to see why these risks may not be increased, as my experience with Gerri demonstrates. Gerri was diagnosed with breast cancer in her late fifties and came to see me with her daughter, Katherine, who was in her late thirties. Gerri expressed concern about her daughter's breast cancer risk, which she estimated as "close to 80 percent." Gerri had four sisters and two brothers, none of whom had been diagnosed with breast or other cancers. Her parents had lived into their eighties without being diagnosed with cancer. None of Gerri's aunts and uncles had a cancer diagnosis, either.

When I told Gerri that her family history was not interesting to a geneticist, she gasped, then laughed, and said she was glad to hear it. However, she added, "I read just the other day that if a woman has a mother with breast cancer, her risk is doubled. Why aren't you interested?"

"You're right," I answered. "As a group, women whose mothers have breast cancer do have twice the risk of women whose mothers don't have breast cancer. But notice, I said *'as a group.'* These studies combine the risk to women whose mother's breast cancer was due to strong hereditary factors with those of women like your daughter, Katherine, whose risk does not appear to be increased as a result of your breast cancer. Some of the daughters have an increased hereditary risk and others do not." I then explained the concept of heterogeneity. Once Gerri and Katherine understood this, they could see how imprecise it would be to base Katherine's risk on a group that included women with very different risks. The point for Katherine is that her mother's family history does not indicate an increased hereditary risk.

Until recently there was no way to distinguish between families that did and did not have breast cancers that were due to strong hereditary factors, so the risks calculated were based on a mixed group of women, only some of whose relatives had hereditary breast cancers. As hereditary factors are increasingly identified, more accurate assessments of risk will be available to women who have affected relatives, as I discuss in chapter 4.

Father's Side of the Family Counts, Too

When I asked one of my patients, a woman named Beatrice, about her father's side of the family she was surprised and said, "My *father* doesn't have cancer." I then explained that information about her father's side of the family is as important as that about her mother's. An increased hereditary susceptibility to breast cancer can be passed through a woman's father as well as through her mother. For this reason, geneticists take both sides of a person's family history into account when they assess risk.

I learned that Beatrice's father's sister was diagnosed with breast cancer in her forties and that his mother and his mother's sister both died of ovarian cancer. Based on this information (and medical records that confirmed the diagnoses) I could tell Beatrice that her father's family history suggested the presence of an increased hereditary risk of both breast and ovarian cancer. There was a 50% chance that her father had inherited a mutation (genetic change) that increased cancer risk. If he had, there was a 50% chance that she had also inherited it (discussed in chapter 3).

Beatrice asked how I determine whether an increased hereditary risk of breast cancer is likely to be present. Her question was an excellent one. Basically, geneticists become more suspicious that strong hereditary factors might be present if an individual is diagnosed with cancer at a young age— say in the thirties or forties instead of sixties. On the other hand, as I discuss in chapter 4, *women with known hereditary breast and ovarian cancers are often diagnosed with cancer after age 50.*

An increased hereditary risk is also more likely if an individual in the family is diagnosed with several different cancers, such as breast and ovarian cancer. Cancer in two or more generations may also suggest an increased hereditary risk, but this is not always the case, particularly with the more common cancers. Also, when three or more close relatives have three or more different types of cancer, the hereditary risk may be increased.

The factors just discussed are listed in the box on page 49. They are a guide, not a rigid set of rules. Some families have several of these elements but the cancers in that family are not hereditary. In other instances, an increased hereditary risk is present but none of these items is present. You will notice how many times I have used the words *may* and *might* in talking about family histories that are likely to suggest increased hereditary risks. I hope this will convince you not to attempt a definitive assessment of your own hereditary cancer risk! To be accurate, assessment of risk is best made by a health professional trained in cancer genetics. I discuss Cancer Risk Assessment at greater length in chapter 9.

Indications That Hereditary Cancers *May* Be Present

- Young age at diagnosis
- One person diagnosed with several different cancers
- Cancers present in two or more generations
- Three or more cancers found in close relatives

Breast Cancer in Men

❧ Few people realize that breast cancer can also occur in men. Male breast cancer is rare, accounting for only about 1% of all cases. In 1999 about 1,000 breast cancers were expected to be diagnosed in men, compared to about 175,000 in women. Countries in which there are higher rates of breast cancer in women tend also to have higher rates in men, compared to countries with lower breast cancer rates for women. And as with women, the risk of breast cancer in men increases with age. In some studies, men who had undescended testes or damage to the testes are found to be at increased risk of breast cancer, compared to men whose testes have not been affected in these ways.

Most breast cancers in men, just as those in women, are not due to strong hereditary factors. *As a group*, men who have a female relative with breast or ovarian cancer do have an increased breast cancer risk. This is a heterogeneous group, so most men whose female relative has breast cancer will never be diagnosed with breast cancer. As noted in chapter 4, men who have a mutation in the BRCA genes are at increased risk of breast cancer.

Key Points to Remember

- The rise in the breast cancer rate in women age 50 and older that occurred from the late 1970s to the 1980s was probably due to increased use of improved early detection techniques.
- The breast cancer rate in women younger than 50 has not substantially increased since the 1970s.

- Geographical differences in breast cancer rates involve very small numbers of women.
- The death rate due to breast cancer has been decreasing since the late 1980s.
- Breast cancers that are found before they measure a little less than half an inch are rarely life-threatening.
- The average woman's risk of breast cancer is 2% from age 20 to 50 and 11% from age 20 to 80.
- Most women who have both a mother and sister with breast cancer are unlikely to be diagnosed with breast cancer.
- An increased risk of breast cancer can be passed through the father's side of the family as well as the mother's.
- You are more likely to find risk information useful and less likely to be misled by it if you:
  - Learn the time over which a risk occurs
  - Avoid comparison risks and look for absolute risks
  - Keep the possibility of heterogeneity in mind.

THREE

☙ ❧

How Cancer Cells Arise

The fantasies inspired by TB in the last century, by cancer now, are responses to a disease thought to be intractable and capricious—that is, a disease not understood—in an era in which medicine's central premise is that all diseases can be cured. Such a disease is, by definition, mysterious.

Now it is . . . cancer that fills the role of an illness experienced as a ruthless, secret invasion—a role it will keep until, one day, its etiology becomes as clear and its treatment as effective as those of TB have become.

—Susan Sontag, *Illness As Metaphor*[1]

As Susan Sontag notes in her book *Illness As Metaphor*, any disease that is not understood "arouses thoroughly old-fashioned kinds of dread." This chapter provides information about the development of cancer cells so that any dread you may have will be removed or lessened. In this chapter you will learn about the role of the genes in bringing about both nonhereditary and hereditary cancers, and how their origins differ. As you will see, it's a fascinating story.

Genes

☙ To understand how cancers develop, you need to be aware of genes, which are composed of long strings of chemicals called DNA, or deoxyribonucleic acid. We are, of course, accustomed to thinking about genes in the eggs and sperm, and their role in reproduction. However, genes are also present in most non-egg and non-sperm cells, which are called so-matic cells.

The genes are wondrous in that they are not only composed of chemi-cals but also make the chemicals that cause our bodies to grow and de-velop. Each chemical produced by a gene must be manufactured precisely. If even one of a gene's chemicals is changed or missing, that gene's product may also have one or more of its chemicals out of place. Such a gene prod-uct may not be biologically active or may not be recognized by the body. You can think of the process as one in which paint is sprayed through a stencil. If the stencil (gene) is ragged or torn, the resulting shape (the chemi-cal made by the gene) may be blurred or illegible.

A change in or absence of one or more of a gene's chemicals is called a mutation. Some mutations are due to accidents in cell division, some to the effects of environmental agents, and some to unknown causes. Damage to the genes in our somatic cells occurs with such regularity that we have a designated team of chemicals whose job it is to move in and repair our DNA.

Chromosomes

The chromosomes are ribbonlike structures that are found in almost every cell of our bodies. Each gene has its own place on its own chromo-some. In figure 4 you will see a photograph of a complete set of human chromosomes as they appear when viewed under a microscope. These chromosomes have been stained to produce the dark and light bands that are used to distinguish one chromosome from another.

Different species have different arrangements of their genetic material. For example, fruit fly genes are contained on only four pairs of chromo-somes, while humans have twenty-three pairs. By convention, chromo-somes are numbered according to size—the two largest are numbers one and two and the smallest are numbers 22 and 23. Figure 5 shows the hu-man chromosomes in order of size from largest to smallest. One chromo-some in each pair is inherited from a person's mother, the other from the father. In figure 5, you will notice that one pair of chromosomes has no number and is labeled with two X's. In humans the chromosomes that determine sex are called X and Y. With some rare exceptions, a woman has two X chromosomes, and a man one X and one Y chromosome.

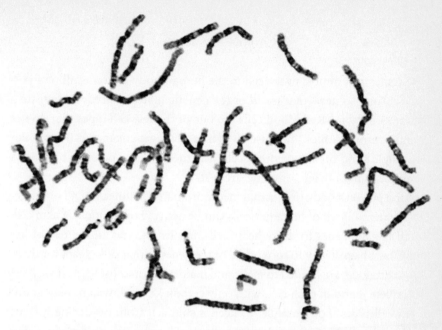

Figure 4. Normal Female Set of Chromosomes (Spread)
Source: Courtesy of Timothy A. Donlon, Ph.D., The Queen's Medical Center, Hawaii.

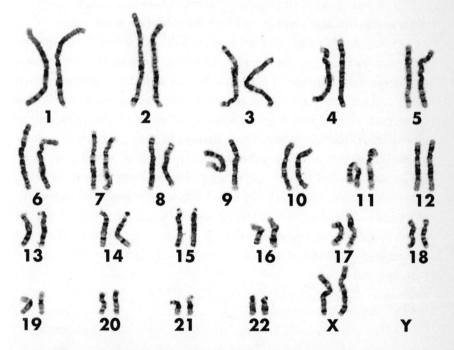

Figure 5. Normal Female Set of Chromosomes (Karyotype)
Source: Courtesy of Timothy A. Donlon, Ph.D., The Queen's Medical Center, Hawaii.

Origins of Cancer

᪥ Amazingly, almost every cell in the human body contains all of a person's chromosomes—that is, *all* of the genetic material needed to create a complete person. (Red blood cells are one of the few cell types that do not contain chromosomes.) Because all of a person's genetic material is present in a single skin, breast, or other cell, it is theoretically possible to grow a complete human being, or clone, from it.

For a person's body to function in a coordinated manner, not all of the genetic material in all of her adult cells can be active. For example, a skin cell, which has the genes to make heart cells, eye lenses, and all the rest of her body, must have a way to turn off all of the genes in that cell except for those whose products are needed to make and maintain skin cells. It's as if we have a complete piano in each cell, with only certain keys allowed to play in different cell types. For example, to keep a skin cell from producing a heart cell's products, "suppressor" or "gatekeeping" genes are needed. In a skin cell these suppressor genes stop non-skin genes from producing their unnecessary and potentially harmful gene products. (Other mechanisms also keep cells in check, but here I will discuss only the role of suppressor genes.)

Cells may divide unless they are stopped from doing so through mechanisms such as the suppressor genes. Therefore, if the suppressor or gatekeeping genes are damaged, a cell might be able to divide in an unregulated manner. As controls are released, more irregular and non-orderly cell division occurs, during which increasingly large parts of the cell's genetic makeup are lost or duplicated. These changes in a cell's genes may eventually enable the cell to develop the capacity to continue dividing in an irregular, uncontrolled fashion and to send cancer cells to other parts of the body (metastasize). Benign (non-cancer) cells have preset times to stop dividing and a defined lifespan. Unlike benign cells, cancer cells have lost the genetic programming that directs orderly division. Signals that tell the cell when to stop dividing and when to die either no longer function or cannot be understood.

Nonhereditary Cancers

Nonhereditary cancers, the majority of all cancers, are due to changes in the genes of a single somatic cell (a non-egg or non-sperm cell), such as a breast cell. You can see now why it is said that all cancers are genetic—they arise when changes occur in the genes of a breast or other cell. But just as important, it is crucial to know that most cancers are not hereditary, because most of the time no changes have occurred in a person's eggs or sperm. Unless a genetic change occurs in an egg or sperm cell, an increased risk of cancer cannot be passed from one generation to another.

Steps leading to the development of a *nonhereditary* colon cancer cell are now known. These cancers arise when mutations occur in at least five different genes in a single colon cancer cell—usually over a period of some years. All of the changes take place after conception—and the changes can occur in different orders. When a sufficient number of braking and organizational mechanisms have been disabled, the cell, in a sense, forgets who it is and where it is and begins the unregulated cell division that we call cancer. Nonhereditary breast cancers are thought to occur in a similar fashion but with changes in other genes.

Some women who are diagnosed with breast cancer search their lives, lifestyle, diet, and emotional state for the cause of their cancer. This was so for Joan, a 53-year-old woman who when I first saw her had just been diagnosed with breast cancer. Joan told me that she was shocked by her diagnosis. "There's none of it in my family and I'm so healthy," she explained. "I've always had a great diet, I exercise, my body is in good shape, I sleep well, Harry and I get along well, and I don't feel angry the way you hear people with breast cancer are." She then added, in a tone of great anguish, "I keep asking myself where I've gone wrong."

To help Joan better understand how a cancer cell can arise, I gave her an example: in some ways the development of cancer is similar to what happens to a rope hanging by a dock. Over time, wind and waves can rub the rope against the dock, enough to wear it away strand by strand. If the wind and waves are strong enough, the rope will eventually break, no matter what its quality. Nonhereditary cancers appear to be due, in many cases, to an interaction between an individual's genes and the environment. A rope hanging by a dock will last longer when the wind and waves are gentle than when they are fierce. In the same way, substances that damage the genes can increase the risk of cancer.

Joan appreciated the explanation about the dock and rope, but perceptively wondered if some ropes were stronger than others.

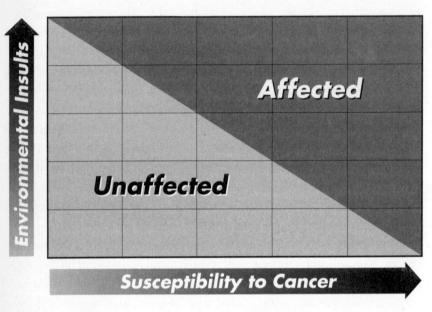

Figure 6. Interaction of Genes and Environment

"I'm not sure about overall strength," I replied, "but different ropes—that is, people—do appear to be strong in different ways." I then asked her to look at a diagram (figure 6), which shows how a person's genes and the environment interact to influence cancer risk. As you can see along the bottom of figure 6, susceptibility to cancer increases toward the right. Along the side, the number of "insults," or changes to a cell's DNA, increases toward the top. Individuals who have a low susceptibility to a particular environmental agent (toward the left at the bottom) can withstand a great deal of exposure to it before one of their cells is damaged enough to escape the normal controls on cell division. On the right side of the diagram are individuals who have such a low threshold of susceptibility to a particular environmental agent that very little exposure may push a cell to the unregulated division, failure to die, and ability to metastasize that we call cancer.

Figure 6 helps to explain why one person who smokes for 50 years does not develop lung cancer, while another, with a different genetic makeup, may develop lung cancer after ten years of smoking. One person's repair mechanisms may be better able than another's to correct any damage to the cell's genes that is brought about by the products in smoke, or one person may be less susceptible to this type of damage than another. From figure 6 you can see why *the* cause of cancer will not be found—there is no single cause. People differ in their genetic susceptibilities to various substances in the environment. These differences in sensitivity are a result of variations in their genetic makeup. Individual differences that are obvious when seen on a case-by-case basis may not be apparent when large numbers of people are studied as a group—another example of heterogeneity, discussed in chapter 2.

Nonhereditary Cancer Recap

Most cancers are not due to strong hereditary factors. They are brought about by changes that occur to the genes in a single somatic (non-egg or non-sperm) cell. All of these changes to the genes in the cell occur *after* conception. Because the changes occur in a somatic cell such as a breast cell, they cannot be passed on to an individual's children. The loss of or damage to several suppressor genes in a single cell can release the brakes on orderly cell division, leading to the development of a cancer cell. Damage to these several genes takes time, so the nonhereditary cancers generally occur at older ages than cancers resulting from hereditary factors.

Environmental agents, accidents in cell division, and failure of DNA repair mechanisms are all thought to contribute to the genetic changes that can lead to the development of a cancer cell. If an individual is susceptible to a particular environmental agent—like radon, for instance—and is exposed to this agent regularly, she is more likely to develop cancer than if she has little exposure. Individuals appear to differ in the ability of their cells to withstand the effects of different environmental agents. Some environmental factors that increase cancer risk, like the effect of asbestos on lung cancer risk, have been identified, but most are still unknown.

If you keep the following points in mind you will find that the distinction between the origin of nonhereditary cancers (presented below) will become clearer to you.

- A person's genes are not confined to egg or sperm cells, but are also present in almost all of the other cells that make up the body (somatic cells).
- Genetic changes that arise in breast or other somatic cells cannot be inherited.
- Genes in cells make the chemicals that cause our bodies to grow and function.
- A change in even one of a gene's chemicals can result in an absent or useless gene product.
- If a gene's product helps to regulate cell division, damage to that gene and therefore to its product may enable the cell to begin inappropriate and disorderly cell division that leads to the development of a cancer cell.

Hereditary Cancers

Unlike the nonhereditary cancers, which arise when changes in *several* genes occur *after conception*, those that are strongly hereditary appear to be due to changes that occur in both members of *a single* very important gatekeeping gene pair. One of the changes is present *at conception* and the other occurs after conception. Hereditary cancers often occur at younger ages than nonhereditary cancers because cancer can arise if only one genetic change happens after conception.

Let's take a closer look. If a woman inherits a mutation in an important suppressor gene from her mother or father, that change is in the egg or the sperm that gave rise to her, and so is present from the moment of conception on. This means that the mutation can be found in all of her cells that contain chromosomes, including her breast cells. With the exception of the genes on the sex chromosomes, we receive two copies of each gene, one from our mother and one from our father. Mutations are rare, so if a woman has inherited a mutation in a strong gatekeeping gene from one parent, the second copy of the gene that she inherited from the other parent probably has no mutation.

The second copy of the important gatekeeping gene, the one that does not have a mutation, appears to be able to produce sufficient gene product to keep the cells in check. However, if at some point after conception it is also damaged or lost, no suppressor gene product will be made. The cell can then escape from control and become a cancer cell.

When I discussed the origin of hereditary cancers with Jane, whose mother and several other relatives were diagnosed with breast cancer, she said, "It looks like my mother might have been born with one of those mutations that she inherited from her father. Then, when she got older, there was another mutation in the second gene like it that she inherited from her mother. After the second gene change, no gene product was made, so that cell became a cancer cell." In Jane's family, this did appear to be how her mother's cancer arose.

When cancers in a family are due to strong hereditary factors, an individual who carries a mutation has a 50% chance of passing on this mutation to each of his or her children. This is shown in figure 7. In the top chromosome pair in figure 7, the chromosome on the left has no gene with a mutation that increases cancer risk, while the one on the right does have such a mutation. In making the egg or sperm cells, only one of each chromosome pair is normally included, so each egg or sperm of an individual who carries a mutation contains either the mutated or the normal copy of that gene. Therefore, each of this individual's children will receive either the chromosome carrying the normal copy of the gene or the chromosome carrying the mutated copy of the gene, as shown in figure 7. The one-out-of-two chance that a mutation will be included in an egg or a sperm results in a 50% chance that each of this individual's children will inherit a particular mutation.

For reasons that are not yet understood, not everyone who inherits one copy of a strong suppressor gene mutation will be diagnosed with cancer. It appears that the second copy of the gene does not always mutate. Factors such as modifying genes at other locations and currently unknown individual or host responses may influence an individual's chances of developing cancer.

Some theorize that instead of being due to changes in the genes, "cancer is a disease that originally occurs at the tissue, rather than the subcellular, level of biological complexity."[2] To date, evidence for the role of genetic changes in the development of cancer cells appears compelling. However,

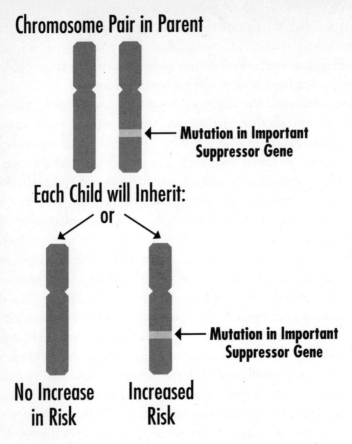

Figure 7. Inheritance of Increased Hereditary Risk

in the future we may well learn more about the role that is also played by what is called the "tissue organization field theory," in which cancer "results from the disruption of cell-to-cell communication."[3] Time and more sophisticated experiments will be needed to determine the role of the "host" or the person in whom cancer develops—and the mutations that help to shape this variability among people. These differences may help to explain why all who inherit a mutation in an important suppressor gene do not develop cancer, or do not do so at the same age.

Hereditary Cancer Recap

Cancers due to strong hereditary factors appear to arise when both members of a strong suppressor gene are damaged or lost. Individuals with an increased hereditary susceptibility have inherited one gene copy in a damaged state (mutation). The second copy of the gene is inherited in an undamaged state. If this second copy is lost or damaged during a person's lifetime—in a breast cell, for example—the cell can no longer function properly. Increasingly unregulated cell growth results, with the cell eventually becoming what we call a breast cancer cell. It's as if there are two red lights at an intersection. If one light is broken, the remaining light is sufficient. However, if the second light is also damaged, no signal remains and accidents may occur.

Important questions still remain. For example, why do some hereditary cancers occur at younger and some at older ages even within the same family? After conception, what causes the normal member of the suppressor gene pair to be lost or damaged? What is the role of environmental factors in encouraging or discouraging a second genetic change? What role is played by other genes or the response of the host (individual carrying the gene)? Scientists who study this area are still working on the answers.

Two Types of Genetic Testing

Unless you remember to distinguish between the terms "hereditary" and "genetic" you can easily become confused by two types of genetic testing. Genetic testing to determine whether an individual has an increased hereditary predisposition to cancer looks for a mutation that was present from the moment of conception. Such a mutation can be found in all of a person's cells that have chromosomes. Genetic testing for hereditary factors is discussed in chapter 4.

A second type of genetic testing is *not* done to determine whether an increased hereditary predisposition is present. Instead, it looks for the presence of genetic changes that have occurred after conception and are *present in cancer cells only*. These two types of testing were confusing to Shirley, a woman without a breast cancer diagnosis who was considering hereditary genetic testing. She called to tell me that her cousin, who had just been diagnosed with breast cancer, was tested for the Her-2 neu gene. "Can you test me for that gene also?" she asked.

I explained that Her-2 neu "overexpression" is a genetic change that is found in about 20% of all breast cancers. These days, when a woman is diagnosed with breast cancer, the breast cancer cells are often tested for the presence of mutations in the Her-2 neu gene (and in other genes as well). When many copies (called overexpression) of Her-2 neu are present in breast cancer cells, the breast cancer is more likely to be aggressive and more likely to have metastasized than if fewer copies are present. Breast cancers that show Her-2 neu overexpression are also more likely to respond to a type of chemotherapy called herceptin than breast cancers with no overexpression.

The point is that Her-2 neu overexpression occurs only in the genes of breast cancer cells. So, in testing for these genetic changes, only breast cancer cells are investigated. It *is* called a genetic test, which leads, understandably, to a confusion between this test and hereditary genetic testing. Her-2 does not appear to be involved in an increased hereditary susceptibility to cancer. It is a good example of a nonhereditary mutation similar to those that occur in the development of nonhereditary colon cancer. Like these, it occurs after conception and is present in the breast cells, not in the eggs or sperm. As a rule of thumb, the aim of genetic tests performed on cancer cells is usually not to detect hereditary mutations. Instead, these tests are designed to look for mutations in cancer cells that can influence an individual's prognosis and treatment.

Key Points to Remember

- All of the genes needed to make an entire person are present in most cells of the body.
- All cancers are genetic, which means they appear to be due to changes in the genes.
- Most cancers are not due to strong hereditary factors. They arise from changes that occur after conception to genes in a single cell in a single organ, such as the breast. Since no genetic changes have occurred in the egg or sperm cells, an increased susceptibility to cancer is not passed from one generation to another.

- Individuals differ in their genetic susceptibility to environmental agents.
- Individuals who have inherited a mutation in an important suppressor gene that increases susceptibility to cancer have a 50% chance of passing that mutation on to each child.
- Not all individuals who inherit a mutation that increases cancer risk will develop cancer.
- There are two kinds of genetic testing:

1. Testing for increased hereditary susceptibility that looks for the presence of a mutation that occurred before conception and is present in all cells that have chromosomes. This mutation increases a person's cancer risk and can be passed on to his or her children.

2. Testing that looks for the presence of a mutation that occurred after conception and is only present in a person's cancer cells. This mutation does not increase a person's hereditary cancer risk and cannot be passed on to his or her children. It can, however, influence cancer prognosis and treatment.

◈◈

FOUR

Genetic Testing for Hereditary Breast Cancer Risk

In this chapter I discuss genetic testing for hereditary breast cancer risk: why people seek testing, the type of risk information that testing provides, testing procedures, interpretation of results, how to identify if you are likely to benefit from testing, and three key elements for you to weigh in making a decision about whether to be tested. This chapter builds on information presented in chapter 3, so you will probably understand the material in this chapter more easily if you read chapter 3 first.

The focus here is genetic testing for the presence of mutations (genetic changes) in two recently discovered genes—Breast Cancer 1 (BRCA1) and Breast Cancer 2 (BRCA2)—and what test results tell us about breast and other cancer risks. I also briefly discuss several other genes for which testing is sometimes considered when an increased hereditary predisposition to breast and other cancers might be present. In chapter 9, I provide guidelines for making a decision about genetic testing and a discussion of some of the social consequences associated with testing.

Why Women Seek Genetic Testing

◈ To appreciate what genetic testing can offer, it's important to realize that before testing was available, if you had concerns about your breast cancer risk due to family history, you would have been able to obtain only the following two types of rather limited information about it:

1. The risk of cancer to women whose family history appears similar to yours. As discussed in chapter 2, women who have a family history of cancer are a heterogeneous group, so your risk could differ considerably from the risk to the group as a whole.

2. The likelihood that your parents carried a mutation that increases cancer risk. If it were likely that one of your parents *did* have such a mutation, there was a 50% chance that you had inherited it and a 50% chance that you had not. There was no way to determine whether you had in fact inherited such a mutation or even to be sure that one of your parents was actually a mutation carrier.

Now, with genetic testing, you *may* be able to learn definitively whether you have or have not inherited a mutation that substantially increases cancer risk. This information can be a tremendous help in planning your health care and in shaping your outlook on life as a whole. However, as I discuss here and in chapter 9, genetic testing is not for everyone, and does not always provide definitive information, even if you have a strong family history of cancer.

Information Obtained in Genetic Testing

As you may remember from chapter 3, genes make the chemicals that are responsible for our body's growth and development. Normally, individuals have two copies of each BRCA gene, with one copy inherited from their mother and one from their father. That is, everyone has two copies of the BRCA1 gene and two copies of the BRCA2 gene. When you hear about "BRCA1 testing" the testing is not done to determine if a BRCA1 *gene* is present, but whether or not the individual has a specific *mutation in one of her BRCA1 genes*. Those who carry a mutation have an increased cancer risk. In the same way, if you hear that Joan "has the BRCA2 gene," it usually means she was found to have a specific *mutation* in one of her BRCA2 genes.

Among the exciting breakthroughs in genetics in the past several years has been the discovery of the exact locations of the BRCA genes. BRCA1 is located on chromosome 17 and BRCA2 on chromosome 13. Now that scientists know where they are located they can investigate these genes for the presence of a mutation that increases cancer risk.

BRCA Mutations and Cancer Risk

℞ Women who inherit a BRCA mutation have an increased risk of breast *and* ovarian cancer. Some are at increased risk of other cancers also, but the greatest risks are for breast and ovarian cancer. To date we know only the approximate cancer risk to someone who has (or carries) a BRCA mutation because:

- Families differ in size. More cancers are likely to be found in a family that has six daughters who live to their eighties than in another family, with the same risk, where there are only two daughters who live to their fifties. With more people in a family who live longer, there is a greater opportunity for cancer to be diagnosed.
- The risk information we now have is largely based on specially selected families in which a number of individuals were diagnosed with cancer, particularly at young ages. Some of the increased cancer risk in these special families may not be entirely due to BRCA mutations, but, for example, to modifying genes that help to increase cancer risk.
- Relatively few women who carry a BRCA mutation have been studied, since genetic-testing techniques are new. With small numbers, the risks are more likely to be influenced by the way in which groups are chosen for study than when larger numbers of individuals are studied.
- The risks of breast and other cancers may be influenced by the location of the mutation within the gene. As you may remember, a gene is composed of many chemicals. If even one chemical is changed or missing, the gene may be unable to make a functioning product. Or if you think of a gene as a building, just as damage to a room near the roof affects a building differently from damage to a room near the foundation, so different mutations may result in different gene products, which in turn influence cancer risk.
- The currently known cancer risks to mutation carriers are based on individuals who carry many different BRCA mutations. This is another example of the concept of heterogeneity discussed in chapter 2. As you may remember, there I pointed out that no matter how carefully you study the contents of a bowl containing several types of fruit, you will not obtain accurate information about only one type.

In the same way, it is important to realize that currently known cancer risks to women who carry a BRCA mutation are based on a collection of different mutations and so are composite risks.

• Some of the currently known risks are estimates and are largely based on the frequency of women with a mutation who develop cancer in both breasts or who develop both breast and ovarian cancer. Factors of which we are still unaware may determine the risk of a second cancer, and the risk of a second cancer may differ from that of a first.

Unless you are aware of the factors that influence the information that is now available for women who carry a BRCA mutation, you may mistakenly believe that these risks are more firmly established than is actually the case.

Breast Cancer

Two of the most commonly quoted studies of risks to women with a BRCA1 mutation are both based on the same 33 specially selected families—families containing many women with breast and ovarian cancer, particularly women diagnosed at young ages. Both studies estimated the breast cancer risk to be about 85% to age 70 in women who had a BRCA1 mutation.[1] A larger study of risks to women with a mutation in the BRCA2 gene was based on 173 families. In this study BRCA2 mutation carriers had a breast cancer risk of 77% to age 70.[2] Many different mutations within the BRCA genes were present in both the BRCA1 and BRCA2 families, and the families were selected for study because they contained many women with breast cancer, particularly women diagnosed at young ages. Therefore, the risk to any one woman who has a particular BRCA mutation or who comes from a different type of family may differ from the risk to the group as a whole. In each study, sizable numbers of breast cancers occurred after age 50.

While the risk to an individual who has a specific BRCA mutation is not currently known with specificity, you can see that as a group, women who carry a BRCA mutation have significantly increased breast risks at older as well as at younger ages. It would be unwise for a woman whose relatives were diagnosed with breast cancer at older ages to assume, based on that circumstance only, that her own hereditary risk is *not* increased.

Ovarian Cancer

As a group, women who carry a BRCA mutation have an increased risk of ovarian cancer as well as breast cancer. One study found a 63% ovarian cancer risk to age 70 for carriers of a BRCA1 mutation.[3] In another study, based on the same group of 33 specially selected families, but using a different method for determining the likelihood that a mutation was present, the risk to age 70 was 44%.[4] The 44% risk of ovarian cancer is more frequently used, since this study's estimates are based on wider criteria for including possible mutation carriers. In a study of 173 families, women who carried a BRCA2 mutation had an ovarian cancer risk of 16% to age 70.[5]

Much of the ovarian cancer risk in BRCA1 and BRCA2 carriers occurred after age 50. These results clearly show that *as a group*, women who carry a BRCA mutation have an increased risk of ovarian cancer, not just breast cancer, and that this cancer often occurs at older ages.

Although BRCA carriers have a lower risk of ovarian cancer than breast cancer, the ovarian risk is in some ways more worrisome. Seventy-five percent of all ovarian cancers have spread by the time they are detected, compared to 38% of all breast cancers.[6] Early detection techniques for ovarian cancer are not very useful, according to a 1994 National Institutes of Health Consensus Development Panel, which stated:

> There is no evidence available yet that the current screening modalities of CA125 and transvaginal sonography can be effectively used to reduce the mortality of ovarian cancer. . . .[7]

The high probability that ovarian cancer will have spread by the time it is detected often leads women who carry a BRCA mutation to consider prophylactic oophorectomy (removal of the ovaries before cancer has been detected). A woman's ovaries can now be removed laparascopically.* Recovery is far shorter than with a traditional hysterectomy. Prophylactic oophorectomy is discussed in chapter 10, along with guidelines for making a decision about this surgery. Hormone replacement therapy, which is generally considered if a woman has her ovaries removed, is discussed in chapter 6.

---

*Surgery with small instruments requiring small incisions. General anesthesia is used, but most women go home the same day.

Risk of Other Cancers

Women who carry a BRCA2 mutation appear to have an increased risk of melanoma, as well as pancreatic, colon, and stomach cancer, but the risk of these cancers is far lower than the risk of breast and ovarian cancer. For example, in one study women with a BRCA2 mutation had about a fivefold increase in pancreatic cancer risk to age 65, compared to women without a BRCA2 mutation. Before you become too concerned about this fivefold increase, please remember the difference between an increase in risk and a high risk, and the lack of useful information to an individual that is often conveyed by a comparison risk, as discussed in chapter 2. In this instance, the fivefold increase in pancreatic cancer risk was an "actual" or absolute risk of 0.7% from birth to age 60 and 1.5% from birth to age 70. These absolute risks are far lower than a fivefold increase in risk might intuitively feel and demonstrate how misleading comparison risks can be. (The average woman's risk of pancreatic cancer is about 0.14% to age 60 and 0.4% to age 70.)

Some, but not most, families with a BRCA1 mutation appear to have an increased risk of colon cancer. Other cancers are found also in these families, but their significance is not yet clear. In families with a BRCA2 mutation, an increased risk of male breast cancer (6% to age 70) is present. Breast cancer has also been found in several men who carry a BRCA1 mutation. Men with a BRCA mutation appear to have an increased risk of prostate cancer.

Risks to Women of Ashkenazi Descent

Many women of Ashkenazi (Eastern European) Jewish descent have heard that their risk of breast cancer is especially high and that BRCA mutations are quite frequent in their ethnic group. In reality, only about 2.5% of individuals of Ashkenazi descent are estimated to carry a BRCA mutation. This means, of course, that more than 97% do not.

Because there has been limited marriage between the Ashkenazi and other ethnic groups, mutations that occurred among the Ashkenazi have tended to remain in that group. When someone of Ashkenazi descent has a BRCA mutation, the mutation is almost always located in one of three specific places. Two of the mutations are in the BRCA1 gene and one is in the BRCA2 gene. Other relatively isolated ethnic groups such as the Icelandics and the Japanese have mutations at other specific locations in the BRCA genes.

In one study, over 5,000 Ashkenazi individuals were tested for the three "Ashkenazi" BRCA mutations. Out of this large number, only 120 were found to carry any one of the three mutations.[8] Women who carried a BRCA mutation had a 56% chance of developing breast cancer up to age 70. The risk of ovarian cancer to mutation carriers was 16% up to age 70.

Before you take these risks too seriously, you need to know that in this study only 27 women who carried a mutation were diagnosed with breast cancer and/or ovarian cancer. And these 27 women carried one of three different mutations. These risks are obviously provisional. Until a much larger number of individuals is studied and risks to those who carry each of the three different mutations is more solidly known, we have only approximate information about the risk of breast and ovarian cancer to a woman of Ashkenazi descent who carries one of them.

Surprisingly, in this study, 26% of those who carried a BRCA mutation had *no* close relative with breast or ovarian cancer. These findings suggest that many people who inherit one of the three mutations may never be diagnosed with cancer or will not be diagnosed until old age. Mutations in genes at other locations may play a role in determining a person's chances of developing cancer when a BRCA mutation is present. Scientists have already located several genes that may do just this.

To avoid the bias of including only individuals who were selected because they had a strong family history of cancer, another study investigated breast cancer risk to Ashkenazi women without regard to their family history of cancer. This study found a 29% risk of breast cancer to age 70 for Ashkenazi women who carry a BRCA mutation—lower than the 56% risk in the previous study but far higher than the average woman's risk.[9]

Several studies have compared the chances of finding a BRCA mutation in young women diagnosed with breast cancer who were and were not of Ashkenazi descent. At each age, Ashkenazi women were more likely to carry a mutation than those of non-Ashkenazi descent. In one study, about 16% of Ashkenazi women diagnosed with breast cancer before age 50 were estimated to carry a BRCA1 mutation, compared to 4% in women in the general population who were diagnosed by the same age.[10] For those diagnosed before age 40, about 27% of the Ashkenazi women were estimated to have a BRCA1 mutation, compared to about 5% in the general population.[11]

As you can imagine, when these risks were reported, many women of Ashkenazi descent were concerned. Some told me that they felt "tainted," "singled out," that they "had weaker genes," and so forth. Actually, when an individual's family history is taken into account, women of Ashkenazi descent are about as likely to carry a BRCA mutation as non-Ashkenazi women. One study compared the chances of finding a BRCA mutation in Ashkenazi and non-Ashkenazi women who had a family history of breast or ovarian cancer and who were themselves diagnosed with breast cancer before 50 or were diagnosed with ovarian cancer. In this study, 43% of the women of Ashkenazi descent had a BRCA mutation, compared to 39% who were not Ashkenazi.[12]

The 4% difference between the two groups may be due to chance, since the number of Ashkenazi women in this study was smaller than the group of non-Ashkenazi women. Also, scientists may be able to find BRCA mutations in Ashkenazi women more easily than in other groups, since almost all Ashkenazi women who have a BRCA mutation will have it at one of three known locations. Other ethnic groups may have a greater proportion of BRCA mutations that cannot yet be found or may have mutations in other, still undiscovered, genes. From the results of this study, you can see that family history appears to be more important than ethnicity in predicting whether a BRCA mutation is likely to be present.

Bilateral Breast Cancer Risks

Women who carry a BRCA mutation are often cautioned about their increased risk of developing a cancer in both breasts (bilateral risk). Their bilateral risk does appear to be increased compared to all women with a breast cancer diagnosis, who have a 0.5% to 1% chance of developing a cancer in the second breast each year. Almost all cancers in a woman's second breast are new cancers that have started in that breast. They are almost never spread from the first breast cancer. That is, they are not a recurrence of the first breast cancer.

Information about the absolute risk of a second breast cancer to women who carry a BRCA mutation is quite preliminary, since it is based on:

- Very small numbers of women with a BRCA mutation who have developed a second breast cancer; for example, in one study the bilateral risks were based on 30 women and in another on only 26—and the women carried different BRCA mutations!

- Women from specially selected research families, whose risks might differ from those of women carrying the same mutation whose family histories of cancer are not as strong.
- Women diagnosed in previous years who were less likely to have as long a survival as that expected in women diagnosed today, and thus would not have as much time to develop a second breast cancer.

For these reasons, the reported bilateral risks to BRCA carriers will almost certainly change as more women are studied.

In one study of nearly 600 women who were carriers of a BRCA2 mutation, 66 developed cancer in a second breast. The chance of developing a second breast cancer was about 2% a year for women diagnosed with breast cancer up to age 50.[13] After age 50 the risk to the opposite breast was about 0.5% to 1% a year—similar to that of all women who had been diagnosed with breast cancer. Studies of women with a BRCA1 mutation, which are based on a smaller number of women, find slightly higher risks.

An earlier study of women who had at least two close relatives with breast cancer but whose BRCA status was unknown found that women who were 50 and older at the time of their first breast cancer diagnosis had about a 1.5% chance of developing breast cancer each year up to twenty years.[14] However, *almost half of this risk occurred in the first five years.* After five years the risk was about 1% a year—no higher than that of all for women with breast cancer.

In these studies of women who had a strong family history of breast cancer, women who were diagnosed with breast cancer before age 50 had a 35% chance of a second breast cancer to twenty years—about 1.75% a year. However, in these women, *a third of the risk (about 12%) occurred in the first five years following their initial breast cancer.* With today's improved early detection techniques, it is likely that many of the breast cancers in these studies that were diagnosed in the first five years would now be found at the time of the first breast cancer diagnosis. In most of today's studies, only second breast cancers found two or three years after the first diagnosis are called bilateral. Those found around the time of the first diagnosis are called "synchronous." I mention this aspect to make you aware of yet another difficulty in applying past study results to women diagnosed today.

If you have a concern about your risk of developing a cancer in the second breast, be sure to learn what your risks are over time, be aware of the limitations of the risks as now known, and remember that *as a woman goes through each year without a breast cancer diagnosis, the risk in that year is left behind.* You can read more about the concept of risk over time in chapter 2. You may also benefit by reading the guidelines for considering prophylactic mastectomy in chapter 10, and by remembering the excellent survival women now have when their breast cancers are found at a small size, as discussed in chapter 2.

Genetic Testing Procedures and Interpretation of Test Results

℞ Now that you have information about the known risks of cancer to women who carry a BRCA mutation, let's turn to the actual testing procedures. Genetic testing for hereditary breast cancer risk usually involves taking a blood sample to examine the genetic material (the DNA which makes up the genes) in white blood cells. Any cell in the body that has a nucleus (those cells that have chromosomes) would do, since a hereditary mutation is present from conception on and so is present in all cells that have a nucleus. White blood cells are generally used since blood is a relatively painless and quick way to obtain a sufficient quantity of genetic material.

At the testing laboratory DNA is removed from an individual's white blood cells, then examined to see if the person's BRCA1 or BRCA2 genes contain changed or missing chemicals. As you may recall, even a small change can result in a gene product that is not useful. The BRCA gene appears to make chemicals that suppress cell division. Therefore, when a BRCA gene product is faulty, it may be unable to prevent a cell from dividing inappropriately, which in turn can lead to the development of a cancer cell.

Although the mechanics of being tested are easy for the individual, the interpretation of test results may be complex. Let's start with those that are straightforward. When the first person in a family is tested, all possible parts of both BRCA genes are investigated to see if a mutation can be found. With some exceptions I'll discuss later, once a mutation is found in that person, other people in the family are checked for the presence *of that same mutation only.* Because mutations are rare, it is unlikely that more than one is present in a family, so subsequent family members are checked only for the presence of the same mutation that was detected in their relative.

When a person is found to have a mutation that increases cancer risk, the result is said to be "positive." A positive result means that the person who carries the mutation has increased cancer risk and can pass the mutation on to her children. As I discussed earlier, each of her children has a 50% chance of inheriting this mutation.

When no mutation that increases cancer risk is found, the result is said to be "negative." A negative result is said to be "definitive" when the person tested has a close relative who is known to carry a mutation that increases cancer risk. For example, if my patient's close relative has a particular BRCA1 mutation, and my patient does not have this same mutation, my patient's negative test result is definitive. My patient is not at increased risk of cancer due to this mutation and cannot pass it on to her children.

What if the first person in the family is tested (all possible parts of both BRCA genes are investigated) and *no* mutation is found? In this case the negative result is not definitive. The person who tested negative may, in fact, not carry a mutation that increases cancer risk. Or she could be carrying a mutation that cannot yet be detected with current techniques.

To make this more clear, you might think of the BRCA genes as buildings and a mutation that increases cancer risk as damage to a room in one of the buildings. As you can see in figure 8, scientists cannot yet enter all of the rooms in the BRCA buildings to look for a mutation. That is, not all of the genetic changes in BRCA genes that increase cancer risk can be detected. And, as you can also see in figure 8, there is some evidence to suggest that there are mutations that increase breast cancer risk in other genes whose location is not yet precisely known. When the precise location of a gene is not known, it's as if the exact street address of that building is unknown, so scientists cannot enter the building to look for damage (a mutation).

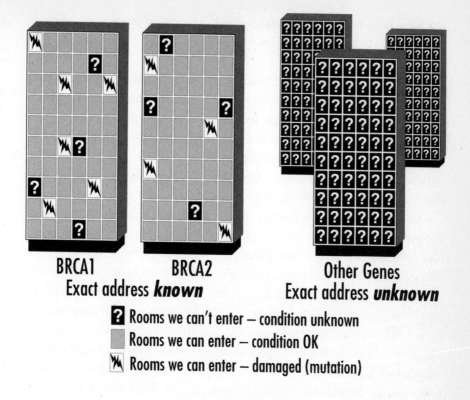

BRCA1
Exact address **known**

BRCA2

Other Genes
Exact address **unknown**

? Rooms we can't enter – condition unknown

   Rooms we can enter – condition OK

W Rooms we can enter – damaged (mutation)

Figure 8. Known and Possible Mutations Increasing Breast
and Ovarian Cancer Risk

You can see that when no mutation is found in an individual, *and there is no known mutation in her close relative*, there are two possibilities: either no mutation is present *or* a mutation is present but it is one that is currently undetectable. In this case, let's assume that my patient's relative is likely to carry a BRCA mutation because of the family history and her relative is the first person in the family who is tested. If no mutation is found, this usually means that no mutation can be detected at present in that entire family. Therefore, it wouldn't make sense to test my patient or her other relatives. Of course, to optimize the chance of finding a mutation, the first person tested is generally someone who has had cancer and who appears, from family history analysis, likely to carry a mutation. In some instances, if one person with a cancer diagnosis is not found to carry a mutation, a second relative who has had cancer and who is also likely to be a mutation carrier may then be tested, since the first person's cancer might not have been hereditary and the second person's might be due to hereditary factors.

Sometimes a woman who has not been diagnosed with cancer has a strong family history of cancer, but none of her affected relatives is alive or none living is available to be tested or wishes testing. In these cases a woman who has not been diagnosed with cancer can still have genetic testing. If the result is positive, the test has shown that she carries a mutation that increases cancer risk. However, if her test result is negative, the result does not mean that no mutation is present. She might carry no mutation *or she might carry one that cannot be found at present.*

One final type of result needs to be considered: a result of "unknown significance." A result is said to have unknown significance when a mutation is found, but scientists are unsure whether this change is one that increases a person's cancer risk. (Not all mutations increase cancer risk. In the analogy of the gene as a building with many rooms, mutations that increase cancer risk are like damaged rooms. Mutations that do not increase cancer risk are like changes in a room. Sometimes testing of several family members will show that the genetic change is present in those who were diagnosed with cancer, but rarely or never occurs in those without a cancer diagnosis. In such cases, the change may then be identified as a mutation that does increase cancer risk. In other instances many individuals without a cancer diagnosis in the family have the mutation, so it is unlikely to contribute to an increase in cancer risk. When it is not possible to trace these changes or to track them sufficiently, the result, for now, remains indeterminate or of unknown significance.

Genetic testing steps for people of Ashkenazi descent differ somewhat, since if a BRCA mutation can be found in these individuals, it will, as discussed earlier, usually be in one of three specific locations. Therefore, in Ashkenazi families, the first person in the family (usually an affected individual) is initially tested for only the three common mutations found in that group. If no mutation is found, full testing of both BRCA genes may be done, since individuals of Ashkenazi descent sometimes (infrequently) carry mutations that are not in one of the three common locations.

When an affected person of Ashkenazi descent is found to have a mutation in one of the three "Ashkenazi locations," that person's unaffected relatives are tested for *all three* mutations, not merely the one found, to rule out the possibility that a second mutation might be present in the family. As discussed earlier, the frequency of BRCA mutations is higher in individuals of Ashkenazi descent than in some other groups, so more than one mutation, while still rare, can occur with higher frequency.

Who Is Likely to Have a BRCA Mutation?

How likely is it that a BRCA mutation will be found in a person's family? Here there are no definitive answers, but we do have some indications of families in which the probability of finding a mutation is higher than in others. As you might expect, women diagnosed with breast cancer at younger ages are more likely to have a BRCA mutation than those diagnosed at older ages. The types of cancers in a family can also provide useful information.

One study investigated the chance of finding a BRCA mutation in women with a family history of breast or ovarian cancer who were themselves diagnosed with breast cancer before age 50 or who were diagnosed with ovarian cancer.[15] As you can see in table 4.1, 31% of the women who were diagnosed with cancer in one breast had a BRCA mutation. About half the women diagnosed with cancer in both breasts or who had a diagnosis of ovarian cancer carried a mutation. Those most likely to have a mutation were women diagnosed with both breast and ovarian cancer—88% of that group. You will notice that except for the last category, approximately half or more in each group did *not* have a BRCA mutation, so mutations in as yet undiscovered genes are probably responsible for many of these cancers.

TABLE 4.1

Chance That Women Diagnosed with Cancer*
Who Have a Family History of Breast or
Ovarian Cancer Carry a BRCA Mutation

Location of Cancer	BRCA Mutation
One Breast	31%
Both Breasts	51%
Ovary	45%
Ovary and Breast	88%

Source: Frank, 1998.

*Breast cancer diagnosed before age 50, ovarian cancer diagnosed at any age.

Some of these categories are based on small numbers, particularly the group that had both ovarian and breast cancer, so the chances of finding a mutation are likely to change as more families are studied.

In some families where many individuals have breast cancer or even breast and ovarian cancer, current testing techniques will be unable to find a mutation. Other families may have only one or two individuals with breast cancer or one with breast cancer and one with ovarian cancer, and a mutation will be found. There are no hard and fast rules, only probabilities. Therefore, it is essential for each person to learn enough to make her own decision about whether she would or would not like to be tested. Aspects to consider when you are making a decision about genetic testing for BRCA mutations are discussed in chapter 9.

Testing beyond the BRCA Genes

⤫ When you hear about genetic testing for increased breast cancer risk, most of the time it's mutations in the BRCA genes that are being sought. However, testing for hereditary breast cancer risk is also available for more rare mutations located in several other genes. Mutations in these genes appear to be responsible for only a small fraction of all breast cancers.

Individuals who have a mutation in a gene on chromosome 10, called PTEN, are said to have Cowden's syndrome. (A syndrome is a group of symptoms or diseases.) In addition to breast cancer, these individuals have an increased risk of thyroid and kidney cancer. Other signs of the syndrome are small raised areas on the face and small growths in the nose, the gastrointestinal system, and on the lips and mouth. Some individuals with this rare syndrome have a large head. Not everyone with Cowden's syndrome will show all aspects of it. Without genetic testing the diagnosis of Cowden's syndrome can be uncertain.

An increased risk of breast cancer is also found in individuals who have another rare syndrome called Li Fraumeni syndrome. Individuals with this syndrome have a mutation in the p53 gene, which is located on chromosome 17. In addition to breast cancer, soft tissue cancers, leukemia, and brain tumors occur. Other cancers are found, but with less frequency. Mutations in p53 are also present in many nonhereditary cancers.

Muir-Torre syndrome, Lynch Syndrome II, and hereditary nonpolyposis colon cancer are syndromes that are all usually due to a mutation in a gene called MLH1, located on chromosome 3, or to one called MSH2 that is on chromosome 2. Individuals with these syndromes are sometimes diagnosed with breast cancer, but ovarian, colon, uterine, and other cancers occur with far greater frequency.

Not all who have a mutation in any of the syndromes just outlined will have all the features of it, nor will all of those who have a mutation in one of these genes develop cancer. *Most individuals whose relatives have one or more of the cancers in these syndromes will not have a mutation in any of these genes, nor will their relatives who have been diagnosed with cancer.* Remember, most cancers are due to nonhereditary factors. For these reasons, I hope you will consult with a health professional who specializes in cancer genetics if you have questions about your family history. I'll tell you how to find these specialists in appendix B. In chapter 9, I discuss what to look for when you visit one.

Who Is Likely to Choose Genetic Testing for BRCA Mutations?

❧ Women most likely to choose genetic testing for BRCA mutations are those who:

- Have a family history of cancer in which there is an increased likelihood that a mutation will be identified
- Can afford the genetic testing fees
- Think that a test result may enhance their emotional well-being or help them to make health care decisions

Individuals differ in their assessment of the importance of each of these areas. Generally speaking, I find that women who have concerns about ovarian cancer risk are more interested in testing than are those who are concerned about breast cancer risk, since breast cancers are far more likely than ovarian cancers to be found before they have spread. I discuss aspects of decision making about genetic testing in chapter 9.

Key Points to Remember

- Assessment of family history cannot detect all the individuals and families who have an increased risk of cancer due to strong hereditary factors.
- Current genetic testing cannot find all the mutations in BRCA and other genes that increase cancer risk.
- As a group, women who carry a BRCA mutation have an increased risk of breast *and* ovarian cancer.
- Currently known risks of breast and ovarian cancer to BRCA mutation carriers are likely to change as more families are studied.
- Women with similar types of family histories of breast cancer or breast and ovarian cancer appear to have the same chance of carrying a BRCA mutation whether they are or are not of Ashkenazi descent.
- Women who inherit a BRCA mutation are often diagnosed with breast and ovarian cancers at older ages, not merely when they are young.
- In one study of individuals of Ashkenazi descent, 26% of those who carried a BRCA mutation had no close relative with breast or ovarian cancer, suggesting that even the taking of meticulous family histories will not identify all who might benefit from testing.
- To determine if current testing techniques can detect a mutation in a particular family, geneticists prefer to test an affected individual in a family before testing those who have not been diagnosed with cancer.
- Three important elements in a woman's decision about whether to obtain genetic testing are: likelihood that a mutation will be found, cost, and whether she thinks the test result will be useful to her emotionally or in planning her future health care.
- Women who have concerns about ovarian cancer risk are more likely to be interested in having genetic testing than are those with concerns about breast cancer risk because breast cancers are far more likely to be found before they have spread than ovarian cancers.

Benign Breast Disease
(The Disease That Isn't)
and In Situ Breast Cancers
(The Cancers That Aren't)

It is our opinion that for the individual patient, a second opinion before a major therapeutic intervention that is predicated
on the pathology results is a valuable exercise that significantly improves care.[1]

Most women, at some time in their lives, have lumps or areas of thickening in their breasts. Some will be told that they have benign breast disease and that no further treatment is needed. Others will have a breast
biopsy (removal of breast tissue) and receive a diagnosis of atypical hyperplasia, ductal carcinoma in situ, or lobular carcinoma in situ.

If the latter is your experience, the very term "diagnosis" may lead you
to assume that a sizable body of scientific information exists about these
entities—and the risk of breast cancer associated with them. In fact, as you
will see, the classifications used to make the diagnoses are not precise. And
information about a woman's future breast cancer risk if she has one of
these cell types is rudimentary, since it is based on studies which generally
have:

- Small numbers of women
- Serious methodological problems
- Different criteria for making diagnoses

Despite these limitations, once a woman is given a diagnosis, the limited information from available studies is often accepted as definitive knowledge.

This chapter is designed to provide a balance to the confidence you may hear expressed about the risks to women who have noninvasive breast changes, and to give you a perspective on the risks that are commonly quoted. Here I will tell you what is actually known about the risks associated with each cell type, and show you why the results of many studies are preliminary. To do this, I will discuss some of the major studies in each area—studies whose results are often used to advise women about treatment. By having information about these studies, you will be able to judge the usefulness of their results in your own situation. I will use terms such as "benign breast disease," "ductal carcinoma in situ," or "lobular carcinoma in situ" because these are the terms you will hear—not because this is the most accurate or useful way to describe the various breast changes.

Although breast cancer risks associated with noninvasive breast changes are not known with certainty, in many situations they appear to be small. So, if you should learn that you have a cell type called benign breast disease or in situ carcinoma, remember that you probably have the luxury of choosing among the options for the treatment that feels right for you, without worrying that you may have jeopardized your life.

Benign Breast Disease

෴ If you have lumps, thickenings, or cysts (fluid-filled sacs) in your breasts, you may have been told that you have "benign breast disease" or "fibrocystic disease." Since most women at some time in their lives have at least one of these changes, the use of the term "disease" is probably a misnomer. In fact a number of investigators have suggested that other terms, such as "lesion," should be used instead of disease, but these have not caught on. Since the term "benign breast disease" is so widely known, I use it in this chapter for changes in the breast that are not invasive breast cancer or in situ breast cancer (see below for a discussion of in situ breast cancer).

Benign breast disease (BBD) is a catchall category that encompasses a number of different changes in breast cells that are brought about by a variety of processes and causes. A woman is usually diagnosed with BBD when cysts, firm areas, or lumps in her breasts are felt. She will, depending on how the areas feel and her own and her doctor's level of concern, either have no further treatment or will have a breast biopsy. If she does have a biopsy the cells in the tissue that is removed are examined under a micro-scope by a pathologist. Criteria used to distinguish one type of BBD from another include the arrangement of the breast ducts, the size of cells and their nuclei, the color of the cell cytoplasm (non-nucleus part of the cell), and the relative proportions of cysts and fibrous tissue.

Most breast cancers are thought to arise in cells that line a breast struc-ture called the terminal ducto-lobular unit, which is part of the breast duct system. In this chapter I will refer to this unit as the duct. The genetic changes that give rise to a nonhereditary breast cancer are less well under-stood than those that produce a nonhereditary colon cancer (see chapter 3). However, it appears that as with colon cancer the breast cells acquire a series of genetic errors that in turn lead to a breakdown of the processes that control a cell's growth, division, and death. These genetic changes can also produce microscopic differences in cell appearance that are seen by the pathologist. The progression of changes in breast cells as now known is shown in figure 9, and is as follows:

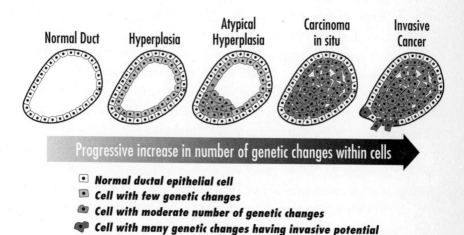

Figure 9. Cellular Changes That Can Lead to In Situ and Invasive Cells

1. Minor changes such as the formation of cysts, which may be due in some cases to genetic changes or to the breast's hormonal environment. Whether the cause is genetic, physiological, or "other," the result is a condition that is called proliferative disease or hyperplasia.

2. Changes in the DNA of a hyperplastic cell produce cells that are enlarged, piled up, and arranged in abnormal complex patterns. These cells are called atypical hyperplasia.

3. Further changes in the DNA of an atypical hyperplasia cell lead to greater abnormalities within the duct. Depending on the pattern of abnormality and its location within a breast duct or a breast lobule, either duct carcinoma in situ (DCIS) or lobular carcinoma in situ (LCIS) cells are formed.

4. Further changes in the DNA of a DCIS cell can lead to the development of an invasive breast cancer. Not all of the DCIS cells become invasive. And not all invasive cancers appear to have a DCIS stage. Furthermore, some scientists believe that changes in an LCIS cell do not directly result in an invasive breast cancer, but that LCIS is a "marker" for increased future risk of invasive disease.

Although these changes are numbered, it's important to realize that cells are by no means destined to make the changes from number 1 to number 2, and so on. They can stop at any stage.

A number of studies have shown that *women with most types of BBD are not at increased risk of breast cancer compared to women without BBD*. In contrast, other well-constructed studies have found that women with BBD have a twofold or even greater increase in breast cancer risk. What accounts for the different results? The answer is heterogeneity, or different types of BBD. Women who have most types of BBD are not at increased risk of breast cancer. However, women with one type, atypical hyperplasia, which constitutes about 10% of all BBD, do have an increased risk, which is far higher than the risk to women who are diagnosed with other types.

A study of breast cancer risk that considers all women with BBD as a single group can obscure the risk to women with atypical hyperplasia and create the impression that all women with BBD have an increased breast cancer risk. For example, if a cup that is 10% filled with red ink (the percent of women with BBD who are diagnosed with atypical hyperplasia) is poured into a cup that is 90% filled with clear water (women with BBD who have no atypical hyperplasia) the full cup of water (all women with BBD) will appear pink. Studies that focus on all women with BBD as a group (the cup filled with pink water) find that all women with BBD have an increased risk. However, there are actually two very different risk groups: women with atypical hyperplasia who are at increased risk and women with other types of BBD whose risk is that of the average woman or close to it. Obviously, when the risk to these two different groups is assessed separately, the results that are obtained are more useful to an individual woman.

Atypical Hyperplasia

As I've discussed, atypical hyperplasia is associated with a higher risk of breast cancer than any other type of BBD. Women with other types have a risk that is not much different from that of the "average" woman. Atypical hyperplasia, like other benign breast "disease" is part of a continuum that passes from "mild and focal" to "marked and extensive." One of the problems with studies on atypical hyperplasia is that there has been little success in determining the risk to women who have the various types, in part because few women have atypical hyperplasia and, of those, even fewer develop breast cancer!

In relative-risk terms, women with atypical hyperplasia have a two- to fourfold increase in breast cancer risk, compared to women in the general population.[2] Now let's consider the absolute (actual) risk, without comparing one group to another. In absolute terms, women with atypical hyperplasia have about a 0.5% to at most a 1% chance of being diagnosed with breast cancer each year. As a woman with atypical hyperplasia goes through a year without developing breast cancer, she leaves behind the 1% or less risk associated with that year. (If you need to refresh your memory of risk over time, you will find this discussed in chapter 2.)

The risks of breast cancer associated with atypical hyperplasia are based on very small numbers of women with this diagnosis who developed breast cancer. One of the largest studies followed 229 women with atypical hyperplasia who had no mother or sister with breast cancer. Over a seventeen-year period, only 22 developed invasive breast cancer.[3] Another study followed 342 women with atypical hyperplasia an average of 21 years. In this time only 33 breast cancers occurred.[4] You can see from the small numbers of women who are diagnosed with breast cancer that the risk is actually quite low. Also, remember that when risks are based on small numbers, they are most usefully viewed as approximations. These risks are likely to change as larger groups are studied.

In one study, women with atypical hyperplasia who had a mother or sister with breast cancer were found to be eight to nine times as likely to develop breast cancer as women in the general population.[5] Some health professionals have used this information as a way to distinguish women with a family history of breast cancer who were most likely to develop breast cancer. Some women have even been encouraged to have prophylactic mastectomy on the basis of these results. As you can imagine, an eight- to ninefold increase in risk was pretty troubling to most who heard about it.

Here again, the number of women studied and the absolute risks can provide some clarity. In one of the largest studies, the risks were based on only 47 women with atypical hyperplasia who had a mother or sister with breast cancer. At the end of twenty years, 12 had developed breast cancer. These women had an absolute breast cancer risk of about 20%—a risk that is no greater than would be expected due to family history alone. (The absolute risk is not the straight percent you would obtain by dividing 12 by 47 since the women were of different ages and not all were followed for twenty years. To take differences in age and follow-up into account, calculations called "life table analysis" are used.)

These risks are also, of course, preliminary. They will probably change as more women are studied and as women with different hereditary susceptibilities to breast cancer are evaluated separately. In absolute risk terms there is no evidence that a woman's risk due to atypical hyperplasia and her risk due to family history can be added together—or that they can be multiplied together as is done in the Gail model. This is a mathematical model for estimating a woman's breast cancer risk. As discussed in chapter 9, it produces overestimates of many women's risks.

If you are diagnosed with BBD, it's important to realize that the highest risk to women with any type of BBD, found in women diagnosed with atypical hyperplasia, is at most 1% a year, and in a number of studies is closer to 0.5% a year. Women with other types of BBD either are not at increased risk or have a risk that is even lower than that of women with atypical hyperplasia.

Ductal Carcinoma In Situ (DCIS)

What Is It, Really?

Ductal carcinoma in situ, also called DCIS and intraductal carcinoma, refers to a group of differently appearing cellular growths that are found in the terminal ducto-lobular unit of the breast. Some of these growths were identified only in the early 1900s,[6] while others were added to the DCIS group more recently. The diagnostic category called DCIS has been associated with uncertainty and even disagreement about its viability as a useful diagnostic category for years. In 1945 researchers declared that the distinction between atypical hyperplasia and DCIS "must be accepted or rejected on grounds of faith in the pathologist or lack of it."[7] Others have referred to the distinction between these categories as "occult." Even in 1998 one investigator asserted that "a vast majority of pathologists" was unable to reliably distinguish between DCIS and some types of benign breast disease.[8] Because the diagnosis of DCIS is made by a pathologist looking at cells through a microscope, "the eye of the beholder" has special meaning here.

There is another issue as well: the name given to the abnormal cells and their growth. Because the term DCIS includes the word *carcinoma*, many women who are told they have these cells understandably assume that they have "cancer" and that their lives are in danger. As I hope you will come to appreciate from the information I present in this chapter, DCIS (and lobular carcinoma in situ or LCIS) are *not* cancers as most of us think of that term. Instead, they are patterns of cell growth that alert us to an increased risk of *future* cancer.

Disagreements between pathologists about DCIS are so great, and the chance that even two well-trained pathologists will make the same diagnosis is so low, that a 1996 article in the British medical journal *The Lancet* was titled "Carcinoma-In-Situ of the Breast: Have Pathologists Run Amok?"[9] The author, who is a pathologist, called for a more relevant classification scheme in order to reduce the fear and confusion that frequently arise when the term *ductal carcinoma in situ* is used. This concern was echoed in the first textbook on DCIS, published only in 1997, in which some experts in the field called for a new classification scheme that "avoids the term carcinoma."[10]

Some progress is being made. In 1997 a consensus panel statement was published with guidelines to establish more consistent diagnoses of BBD and noninvasive diseases. Even more precise diagnoses will be possible when it becomes possible to go beyond a cell's appearance under a microscope and directly detect various genetic changes in the in situ cells. Then it will be possible to learn which cells tend to become a cancer, which do not, and which are "marker cells" that indicate a woman has an increased risk, but do not become cancer cells themselves.

Why are investigators concerned about the classification and naming of DCIS? Why do they feel the word *carcinoma* in the term *ductal carcinoma in situ* can be misleading? The answer is that to most of us, a cancer is a tumor or growth that can send cells into the adjacent tissues (invasion) and to other parts of the body (metastasis). The most feared outcomes of breast cancer result from its metastatic behavior. A cancerous tumor of the breast can metastasize to other organs, while a non-cancerous tumor, no matter how large, cannot. The fact is *DCIS cells lack the biological capacity to metastasize*. Because carcinoma in situ neither invades nor metastasizes, some have pointed out that the term *ductal* carcinoma *in situ* is an oxymoron—a cancer that doesn't do what cancers do! As you saw in figure 9, DCIS cells can develop into invasive cancer cells. But then, so can most cells in the body, given enough genetic changes. (To read more about these changes, see chapter 3.)

Even though DCIS cells have some of the microscopic features of invasive cells, they have not penetrated the lining of the duct in which they arise and grow. You can see the change from DCIS to invasive carcinoma in figure 9. Here it's important to realize that DCIS cells do not burst from a duct when the duct is filled. Instead, a change must occur in a DCIS cell to transform into one that has the capacity to go through the duct wall and to survive in the connective tissue of the breast.[11] Before DCIS cells can become invasive and gain the ability to leave the duct, genetic changes must occur in them. Therefore, the use of the term *carcinoma* to label cellular abnormalities within a duct can be misleading.

The inability of DCIS to metastasize became apparent in the 1980s when 100 women with DCIS had the lymph nodes under their arms examined and no cancer cells were found in them.[12] In a more recent report of 319 women with DCIS, only two had lymph node metastases.[13] In these two women, the metastases were probably due to the spread of cells from an undetected invasive cancer that was also present in the breast, but was not detected by the pathologist.

A recently developed method makes it possible to find even a few cancer cells in lymph nodes under the arm—cells that could not be detected with methods used a few years ago. The biological importance of the presence of a very small number of cancer cells in the lymph nodes does not appear to be associated with future risk of cancer in other parts of the body. However, their significance is currently unknown and will await long-term studies. As I discuss in this chapter, women with DCIS almost never develop metastatic disease when:

- Their breasts are carefully examined for the presence of invasive breast cancer and none is found.
- They have complete removal of their DCIS.

These studies show that DCIS does not have the ability to send cancer cells beyond the lymph nodes to other parts of the body. Only invasive cancer cells appear to have this ability.

Frequency of DCIS

DCIS may occur in a woman's breast as the only abnormality or may be found when an invasive breast cancer is diagnosed. This chapter discusses *only* DCIS that is *not* associated with invasive disease. (When both DCIS and invasive breast cancer are found in the same breast, the treatment and chances of recurrence in the breast or spread to other parts of the body are a function of the *invasive* disease, not the DCIS.)

DCIS has been found with increasing frequency in recent years as more women have had mammograms, as mammography techniques have improved, and as pathologists have come under increasing pressure to recognize and label the earliest changes that can in time lead to a breast malignancy. DCIS now accounts for 30% to 40% of all new so-called breast cancers.

DCIS can sometimes be felt, but these days it is usually found when a breast biopsy is recommended for a woman whose mammogram shows abnormalities, such as irregular clustered micro-calcifications. These calcifications can arise when the death of DCIS cells alters the acid-base ratio in that part of the breast duct, causing calcium salts that are normally found in the blood to be attracted to the site of the chemical change. This calcium provides a visual marker when a woman has a mammogram. However, not all calcifications are due to DCIS, nor does all DCIS result in the formation of calcification.

Natural History of DCIS

Some women probably have DCIS that is not detected on a mammogram or felt during a physical examination and never develops into invasive cancer. Autopsy studies of women in whom neither invasive breast cancer nor DCIS was suspected have found that 4% to 15% of the breasts examined contained DCIS cells.[14] As you might expect, the chance of finding DCIS in these women's breasts increased dramatically as larger amounts of breast tissue were examined by a pathologist.

The results of the autopsy studies suggest that DCIS can remain as DCIS without becoming invasive, or can remain as DCIS for a long time. These findings are supported by a study of living women. In this study, breast tissue was reexamined some years after a group of women had surgery for non-cancerous breast conditions. In 60 of these women DCIS was initially overlooked, so they received no treatment other than a breast biopsy. Of these 60 women, about 25% developed an invasive breast cancer in the fifteen years after their surgery.[15] This means, of course, that 75% of the women never developed breast cancer.

Much of the overlooked DCIS in this study was the type that is least likely to recur, so these results do not apply to women with other types of DCIS, as I discuss later in this chapter. If you are diagnosed with DCIS, don't be lulled into thinking it can be ignored. When DCIS is found, it needs to be treated, since there is at present no way to tell which DCIS will become invasive over time and which will remain DCIS. However, as you will see, it is clear that some types of DCIS are more likely than others to become invasive.

You may hear DCIS referred to as a "precancer." I find that this term is not useful and may even be confusing. When many people hear "precancer" they quite reasonably think it means that a cell is *definitely* on its way to becoming a cancer—perhaps tomorrow. Actually, as the studies reviewed above report, a DCIS cell does not always become invasive. If it does become invasive, it generally takes months or years to do so. Since we don't know which cells will eventually become cancer cells, and since almost any cell in our bodies has the potential to accumulate the genetic changes needed to become a cancer cell (see chapter 3), the term "precancer" could be applied to most cells! The presence of DCIS is probably most usefully viewed as an indication that a woman's risk of a future breast cancer is increased, particularly if she receives no treatment for it. *If she has effective treatment, many studies find that for most women with DCIS the chance of developing invasive breast cancer is no greater than if she were diagnosed with atypical hyperplasia—a risk of about 1% a year.*

When DCIS Is Diagnosed

If you are told that DCIS cells were found in your breast biopsy, be assured that you have months in which to learn enough to be able to make the decisions that are right for you—without in any way endangering your life. In addition to using some of the information presented in Part III of this book, you may find that your decision-making process will be more effective if you obtain answers *that make sense to you* about the following five questions:

1. What is it?

2. What size is the DCIS that was found in my breast?

3. How close is the DCIS to the margins of my biopsy?

4. What type of DCIS is it?

5. What are the treatments available and the chance of recurrence* after each type of treatment?

I discuss each of these questions in the sections that follow.

What Is It?

There is an important difference between duct carcinoma in situ and invasive breast cancer cells, even though the term *carcinoma* is used. Unless you understand the distinction between invasive and in situ carcinoma, you may mistakenly assume that you are at high risk of developing

---

*In this chapter, *recurrence* refers to future development of either more DCIS or invasive breast cancer in the same breast in which the DCIS was found—*not* elsewhere in the body.

cancer in other parts of your body—an ability that DCIS cells lack. You will probably find it useful to obtain a pathology reading and written report from a pathologist *who has expertise in the area of DCIS*. When you do, it is important to realize that the pathologist must balance various criteria seen in the cells in assigning a diagnosis. Some pathologists make a diagnosis on very subtle changes, while others may require more changes to make the same diagnosis. *All* of the breast tissue removed must be carefully examined to be sure that a small amount of invasive breast cancer is not present. If you are found to have even a small amount of invasive breast cancer along with DCIS, the rest of this chapter does not apply to your situation.

Be sure you receive a copy of your pathology report (or reports) and have one or more of your physicians review it with you. From the report you should be able to learn:

- The size of the DCIS
- An assessment of the tissue around the DCIS (the margins), particularly:
  - Whether a rim of uninvolved tissue is present around all of the DCIS
  - The size of the clear tissue around the DCIS
  - The type or types of DCIS that are present

If you are not clear about these issues after reviewing your pathology report, you may need another reading by a pathologist who can provide these answers, or more visits to discuss the pathology report you have. If the pathologist does not practice in a setting where biopsies of this type are an everyday event, then it is almost always a good idea to get a second pathology opinion.

If you had a biopsy because calcifications were present in one part of your breast, you will also want to be sure that *all* of them were removed during the biopsy. An X ray of the tissue that was removed, called a "specimen mammogram," should show the presence of the calcifications that were seen in the mammogram you had before your surgery to remove the DCIS. You will need to have another mammogram of your breast when it is healed so you can be absolutely sure that no calcifications (and perhaps more DCIS or even a small amount of invasive breast cancer) remain.

What Size Is It?

To make an informed decision about treatment for DCIS, you will want to know how likely it is that more DCIS or invasive cancer is present in another part of your breast. If you have DCIS in only a single, small part of your breast, that DCIS and a small area of uninvolved tissue around it (called a clear margin) can usually be removed. The surgical removal may be called an excision, a biopsy, or a lumpectomy. All three of these terms refer to surgical removal of tissue. If you have a small amount of DCIS, this one surgery may be the only treatment you will need. If several different areas of your breast contain DCIS or if invasive breast cancer is present, you will need more treatment.

The size or the extent of the DCIS is a most important consideration. As the size of DCIS increases, so does the likelihood that other parts of the breast contain either more DCIS or invasive breast cancer. Put positively, the smaller the DCIS the less likely it is that any other part of your breast is affected and the more secure you can feel about having treatment only to the part of the breast in which the DCIS is found. Also, as a generalization, the smaller the size of the DCIS, the lower the chance of recurrence will be.[16]

Because DCIS is often not visible to the pathologist except when viewed under the microscope, and because the DCIS may be irregular in shape, it can be difficult to obtain an exact measurement of it. In one careful study, women whose DCIS was more than 56 millimeters (mm) in size had invasive breast cancer in another part of their breast nearly half the time.[17] In those whose DCIS measured less than 56mm and who had their DCIS completely removed, no invasive breast cancer was found elsewhere in the breast.

What Size Are the Margins?

Margin size, or the area of clear tissue around the DCIS, appears to be one of the most important predictors of whether DCIS or invasive cancer will develop in a woman's breast after treatment for DCIS. With a larger rim of uninvolved tissue, the chance of recurrence is lower because there is a greater likelihood that all of the DCIS has been removed.[18] In a number of studies in which the location of a recurrence within the breast was noted, almost all were found at or very close to the site of the original DCIS, suggesting that they arose from DCIS cells that had been unknowingly left behind.[19] If you think of DCIS cells as snake eggs, you can see why removal counts. If all the eggs are removed, no snake can emerge to bite you. That is, no more DCIS or no invasive cancer can develop because no eggs remain.

One careful study assessed margins of different sizes and the likelihood of recurrence up to 8 years. Women who had a margin of 1 cm (a little less than half an inch in size) around their DCIS almost never had a recurrence. When the margin was smaller, the chance of recurrence increased.[20] For this reason, the margins should contain no DCIS or invasive cancer and be as large as possible—at least 1 mm and preferably 1 cm. As the distance between the DCIS and the surgical margin of the tissue that was removed becomes narrower and narrower, the probability that there is an area of undetected DCIS remaining in the breast becomes greater and greater.

What Type Is It?

There are different types of DCIS, some of which recur with greater frequency than others. However, there is as yet no agreement among pathologists about how to classify these different types. It is an evolving process. Because of the lack of agreement, investigators classify different types of DCIS having different probabilities of recurrence in different ways, making it difficult to compare the results of one study with those of another.

Progress is being made, however. A 1997 consensus statement by a group of eminent pathologists has helped to encourage use of the same criteria in making diagnoses. Increasingly pathologists are classifying DCIS by the appearance of cell nuclei and the presence or absence of cells that have died, a process called necrosis.[21] When abnormal looking cell nuclei and necrosis are present, a recurrence is more likely than when these features are absent. The most widely used classification, called the Van Nuys Grading Scheme, uses the appearance of nuclei and the presence or absence of necrosis to divide DCIS into three types, with Group I having the least likelihood of recurrence, Group II an intermediate likelihood, and Group III the greatest.[22]

One study investigated the risk of recurrence to women with each of the three types of DCIS. I've listed the results of this eight-year study in table 5.1. You can see that women with Group I DCIS had a 7% chance of recurrence. The recurrence risk for those with a Group II DCIS was 16%, while those with Group III DCIS had a 39% chance of recurrence at eight years. About half the recurrences were DCIS and half invasive disease. In each of these three groups women received different treatments. Some were treated with surgical removal alone,* some with surgical removal plus radiation therapy, and some underwent mastectomy.

In table 5.1, you can see that women with Group II DCIS had larger amounts of disease than did those with Group I. Women with Group III DCIS, who had the highest rate of recurrence, also had the most extensive disease. You may remember that as the size of DCIS increases, hidden invasive cancer is more likely to be present. Also with larger size the margins are likely to be smaller, because the surgeon is attempting to provide a woman with a good cosmetic result. (The more breast tissue removed, the greater the chance that the appearance of the breast will be altered.) With small margins, as I reviewed above, the risk of recurrence also increases. These factors, as well as the type of DCIS, probably contributed to the higher rates of recurrence in Groups II and III when compared to Group I.

TABLE 5.1

Type of DCIS and Chance of Recurrence to Eight Years

Group (Type of DCIS)	Number of Women	Average Size	Chance of Recurrence[†]
I	139	20 mm	7%
II	157	24 mm	16%
III	129	37 mm	39%

Source: Silverstein et al., 1995.
[†]Half were DCIS and half were invasive breast cancer.

What Are the Treatments and Recurrence Rates?

After receiving a diagnosis of DCIS the options available to you may seem bewildering: mastectomy, surgical removal, surgical removal plus radiation therapy, or tamoxifen. Sorting through these options can seem arduous. As Francine said, "I feel as if all this decision making is driving me a

---

*In this and other sections "surgical removal" refers to removal of the DCIS, not the breast. I have reserved the term mastectomy for removal of the entire breast.

little crazy at times." Many women tell me they have the urge to do "something, anything, just to get back to my old life." They can't, of course, go back to their old life as it was before their diagnosis. Experiences since then have changed them and often their perspective on mortality, on the medical profession, and even on their relationships with others. They can, however, fashion a new life that is full, joyous, and long-lasting. If you are diagnosed with DCIS you are more likely to be pleased with the treatments if you take time to be sure you are making decisions that are right for you. To do so, you need to make decisions based on information, not fear.

It's important to realize that you have a variety of options after a DCIS diagnosis because "real" cancer isn't present, nor has a spread occurred from these cells to other parts of your body. There are several ways to treat abnormal cells in the breast or, as the doctors say, "locally control" DCIS. One way is mastectomy. A woman who has a mastectomy to treat her DCIS has about a 3% chance of a recurrence in that breast in the next ten years. If you have a large amount of DCIS you may be more likely to decide to have a mastectomy than if a small amount is present, especially if adequate removal of all the DCIS would entail also removing most of your breast.

In this section I focus on some of the larger and longer-running studies that have examined a woman's chance of recurrence after a diagnosis of DCIS—studies you are most likely to hear about from your doctors. I have used these studies to illustrate some of the issues that may be useful to you in making a treatment decision. This is an area in which new information is becoming available all the time, so be sure to ask your doctors about the results of the latest studies. Then, use the tools in this book to analyze them. Be sure to apply the questions posed in the section "When DCIS Is Diagnosed" to these new studies.

Initial Landmark Study

Until 1982, women who were diagnosed with DCIS routinely received a mastectomy. A landmark study published at that time showed that women who had small amounts of DCIS were unlikely to have a breast recurrence when all of the DCIS and a small amount of normal tissue around it was removed.[23] Women who had larger amounts of DCIS were less likely to have all of the DCIS completely removed and were therefore also more likely to have a recurrence. About half the recurrences were DCIS and half invasive disease. Even so, the women in this study did not develop widespread breast cancer and did not die of it.

Since this landmark study, others have confirmed its findings—that mastectomy is generally no more useful than more limited surgical removal in treating DCIS, unless the DCIS is quite extensive. The primary issue for many women with a DCIS diagnosis has changed from whether to have a mastectomy to whether they are likely to benefit from radiation therapy or from tamoxifen after their DCIS is surgically removed.

Large National Study Using Radiation Therapy

B-17, a large national study, compared breast cancer recurrences in over 400 women whose DCIS was treated by surgical removal alone with recurrences found in over 400 women who were treated with surgical removal followed by radiation treatment.[24] I've listed these results in table 5.2. You can see that over an eight-year period the women who were treated with surgical removal had only a 13% chance of developing *invasive* breast cancer, compared to a 4% chance for those who received radiation therapy. The chance of developing *noninvasive* disease (either DCIS or LCIS) was 13% for women who had no radiation therapy and 8% for those who received it.

TABLE 5.2

Eight-Year Breast Recurrence for
Women Whose DCIS Was Treated with Surgery
Only or Surgery and Radiation Therapy

Type of Breast Recurrence	Surgery Only	Surgery and Radiation Therapy
Invasive	13%	4%
Noninvasive	13%	8%
Total	26%	12%

Source: Fisher et al., 1998.

Because the women who were treated with both surgical removal and radiation therapy had less chance of recurrence than those treated with surgical removal only, some health professionals concluded that *all* women with DCIS would benefit from radiation treatment. Here an investigation into the way in which this study was constructed and conducted may lead you to conclude, as I did, that much or all of the difference in risk between the women who did and did not receive radiation therapy may well have been due to study methodology, not to the radiation treatment they received.

One of the major and most unfortunate aspects of this study was the failure to obtain a pathology review on over a quarter of the biopsies. Even when tissue was reviewed, not all of it was examined. Unless all of the tissue is examined, there is no way to be sure how large the DCIS was or that invasive disease was not also present. If women with invasive cancer *were* unknowingly included in this study, we would expect fewer invasive recurrences in those who received radiation therapy, since radiation therapy has long been found to help control invasive disease.

If radiation therapy were more effective in treating invasive breast cancer than in treating DCIS, we would expect that women who received radiation therapy would have a greater reduction in invasive disease than their DCIS rates. In fact, this is what table 5.2 shows. Invasive breast cancer was less likely to occur in women who received radiation therapy, compared to those who did not—a 9% difference. Radiation therapy was less successful in reducing the risk of noninvasive disease—a 5% difference. This finding suggests that radiation treatment may be less effective in treating noninvasive than invasive disease. More studies will be needed to confirm this.

The supposition that women with invasive breast cancer were included is supported by the presence of 14 women in this study who died of breast cancer over a period of eight years. Four of them had surgical removal alone and 10 had both surgical removal and radiation treatment. No other large study of DCIS has had so many women die of breast cancer, since DCIS does not metastasize. In fact, the presence of the unexpectedly large number of women with metastatic breast cancer makes it quite likely that many, many women with invasive breast cancer were included in this study. It is highly unlikely that any of these women developed invasive breast cancer after their DCIS diagnosis and entry into the study, since invasive breast cancer generally takes more than eight years to grow before it can be detected.

According to one investigator, this national study was "in some respects . . . a giant leap backward in the study of DCIS" because of its methodological flaws.[25] Other researchers point out that when the national study began, different types of DCIS were not as clearly understood as they came to be in the 1990s.[26] These investigators called for future national studies to include the following in their methodology:

- Careful measurement of the extent of a woman's DCIS
- Complete investigation of *all* breast tissue removed
- Clear margins around the DCIS
- Measurement of margin size
- Classification of DCIS by type

If these elements are included in future studies, it will be possible to determine which groups of women with DCIS might benefit from radiation therapy and which will do well with surgical removal of their DCIS without further treatment. Please look at table 5.2 once more. You will see that for women whose DCIS was treated with surgical removal only, there is at most a 13% chance of developing invasive breast cancer spread over eight years. This is about 1.6% a year—a risk that might well be smaller if the methodological issues just discussed had not been present. One further point: the total 26% chance of a breast recurrence at eight years is higher than almost every other published study on DCIS. The other studies were smaller and were usually conducted at only one or two institutions, so the researchers had more control over the quality of the pathology review and the size of the margins that were obtained at surgery—two factors that were not well controlled in this study and that probably contributed to the higher overall recurrence rate.

Van Nuys Prognostic Index

In an attempt to make DCIS treatment decisions easier, one group of investigators devised what they call the Van Nuys Prognostic Index (which should not be confused with the Van Nuys Grading Scheme for classifying the different types of DCIS described above). The Prognostic Index uses a scale to rate each of the following: size of the DCIS, size of clear margin around the DCIS, and type of DCIS.[27]

When this scoring system was applied to a group of women with DCIS who were followed for twelve years, those whose DCIS had the lowest score were least likely to have a breast recurrence, those with intermediate scores were more likely to recur, and those with the highest scores had the highest rates of recurrence.[28] In table 5.3 you can see that when the score was 3 or 4 (the lowest category), none or almost none (0 to 3%) of the women had a breast recurrence, whether they had radiation treatment after surgical removal or were treated with surgery only.

TABLE 5.3

Van Nuys Prognostic Index and Twelve-Year Breast Recurrence Rates*

Index Score	Number of Women	Average Size	Surgery Only	Surgery Plus Radiation Therapy
3–4	116	8 mm	3%	None
5–7	245	16 mm	36%	26%
8–9	33	38 mm	100%	62%

Source: Silverstein and Lagios, 1997.
*About half were DCIS and half invasive disease.

Women whose DCIS was in the intermediate category (5 to 7) were more likely to have a recurrence than those whose score was 3 or 4. In this intermediate group women were less likely to have a breast recurrence if they received radiation treatment. At the end of twelve years, 36% of this group treated with only surgical removal had a recurrence, compared to 26% for those who had both surgical removal plus radiation therapy. Women whose DCIS had the highest scores (8 and 9), also had the highest rates of recurrence. In this group, all of the women who were treated with surgical removal alone had a recurrence. Even with radiation treatment the rate of recurrence in this group was high: 62%.

Some health professionals who read this study decided that if a woman's DCIS had a score of 3 and 4 she should be treated with surgical removal of the DCIS only. Those whose DCIS had scores 5 through 7 should have surgical removal plus radiation treatment and those with scores of 8 and 9 should have a mastectomy. By adding up the numbers, decision making could be quick and easy. These individuals ignored or did not realize that the authors of the study suggested that the scores be used as an *adjunct* in discussing treatment, especially for women whose DCIS had a score of 5 to 7.

Let's take another look at table 5.3. You can see that as the Index score goes from 3–4 up to 8–9, the size of the DCIS also increases. With increasing size, the margin of clear tissue around DCIS often decreases, since the size of women's breasts is limited, as discussed earlier. Also, as DCIS size increases, so does the likelihood that hidden invasive disease is present or that positive margins have been overlooked, leaving DCIS in the breast after surgery. These factors also increase the likelihood of recurrence. In women whose DCIS had a 5 to 7 score, note also that the chance of invasive breast cancer differed by very little regardless of treatment—about 1.5% a year for women treated with surgical removal alone (18 ÷ 12 = 1.5% per year) and about 1% a year for women receiving surgical removal and radiation therapy (13 ÷ 12 = 1% a year). Remember, half the recurrences were invasive. As a woman goes through each year without a diagnosis of breast cancer, she leaves that risk behind.

If you are asked to make a treatment decision based on the Van Nuys Prognostic Index, or if you learn that your doctor is basing his or her treatment recommendation on this Index, remember that this approach *combines* size of DCIS, margin size, and type of DCIS. In your particular case, one of these elements might be of particular importance—for example, having a type of DCIS that rarely recurs or having a small amount of DCIS with margins that are not clear.[29] Margins are particularly important, as you will see in the next section.

Margin Size: A Recent Study

A 1999 study investigated the effect of margin size on recurrence in women with DCIS who were treated with either surgical removal alone or surgery followed by radiation treatment.[30] (Margin size is the amount of healthy tissue around the DCIS that is surgically removed.) Table 5.4 shows the results of this eight-year study. You can see that when the margins were large (10 mm+), radiation treatment did not appreciably reduce the very low recurrence rate of 3%. In fact, without radiation therapy, the risk was slightly lower. As the margin size decreased, however, the risk of recurrence increased, *with and without radiation treatment.* When the margin was between one and 10 mm, there was a 20% chance of recurrence without radiation treatment, compared to 12% if radiation treatment was used. When the margins were very small, there was a 58% chance of recurrence without radiation and a 30% chance with radiation.

TABLE 5.4

Margin Size and Eight-Year
Recurrence* after DCIS

Margin Size	Surgery Only	Surgery and Radiation Treatment
10 mm+	3%	4%
1–10 mm[†]	20%	12%
Less than 1 mm[‡]	58%	30%

Source: Silverstein et al., 1999.
*Includes both DCIS and invasive breast cancer.
[†]Difference is not statistically significant and so is more likely to be due to other factors, not the treatment.
[‡]Difference is statistically significant, and so is more likely to be due to the treatment.

This study shows the great effect that margin size has on the likelihood of a future breast recurrence. A small margin size (a small amount of clear tissue around the DCIS) means it is more likely that some DCIS had been inadvertently left behind. The larger the margin, the lower the chance of recurrence. Even when the margins are very small, women who receive radiation treatment *still* have a higher rate of recurrence than women whose margins are larger and who have no radiation treatment. *Radiation therapy does not appear to make up for the lack of a clear margin.* In this study, as in several others, about half of the recurrences were invasive and half DCIS. With adequate margins, margins of 1 mm to 10 mm, the risk of invasive disease was 1.3% a year with surgical removal and 0.8% with surgical removal plus radiation therapy. This difference is not statistically significant, and so is most likely due to factors other than treatments. (For a discussion of statistical significance, see chapter 6.)

The results of this study, by the same group that developed the Van Nuys Prognostic Index, raise further questions about the advisability of using the Index as a primary treatment-decision tool. Instead of relying on radiation treatment if the margins are small, you may want to discuss the possibility of having more tissue removed to obtain margins that are greater than 1 mm in size and preferably 1 cm in size, regardless of the extent or type of DCIS. Remember that a millimeter is less than 1/16 of an inch, leaving very little room for error. As you can see, when the margins are 1 mm or less, the risk of developing invasive breast cancer in the future is high, *even when radiation therapy is used.*

Throughout this section I have mentioned the future risk of developing invasive breast cancer—a risk of less than 1% to 1.5% a year for many women with a DCIS diagnosis. It is instructive to compare this risk to the risk of invasive disease for women who are diagnosed with atypical hyperplasia. You may remember that women with atypical hyperplasia have a risk of invasive breast cancer of 0.5% up to 1% a year. These women do not usually have their breast removed, nor are they treated with radiation therapy.

By comparing the up to 1% risk a year after a diagnosis of atypical hyperplasia with the 0.8% to 1.3% a year risk of invasive breast cancer to women with DCIS who have adequate margins, and who are treated by surgical removal alone, you may have a different perspective on your risks after a DCIS diagnosis. You may find, as many women do, that treatment recommendations for DCIS are often driven by the name given to the cell, not by the increased chance of developing invasive breast cancer in future, that accompanies it. This is particularly the case for small, low-grade DCIS that has been completely removed.

Tamoxifen for DCIS?

B-24, another large national study, compared risk of invasive recurrence in women with DCIS who were and were not treated for five years with tamoxifen (a drug frequently prescribed for women with invasive breast cancer to reduce risk of recurrence in the breast and elsewhere in the body). In this study, all of the women had surgery to remove the DCIS as well as radiation treatment after their surgery. Half of the 1,798 women then received tamoxifen for five years and half did not. To enter this study *a woman did not have to have all the DCIS removed, nor was all of the tissue examined after it was removed.*

Unsuspected, small amounts of invasive cancer were probably present in a number of the women who participated, since four in one group and two in another developed cancer in the chest wall or lymph nodes under the arm during the five years of the study.[31] Invasive cancer takes longer than five years to develop and be detected, so these cancers were almost certainly present before the study began.

At the end of five years, about 4% of the women who did not take tamoxifen and 2% of those who did developed an *invasive* breast cancer. About 5% of the women who did not take tamoxifen and 4% of those who did developed more *noninvasive* disease (either DCIS or LCIS). These risks are shown in table 5.5. As you can see, for invasive breast cancer there is a 2% difference in risk between those who did and did not take tamoxifen—a difference of about 0.4% a year. Another way to view these findings is to realize that *53 women would need to be treated with tamoxifen for five years before one less case of invasive disease would be found, compared to a group of women who were not taking tamoxifen.* No difference in breast cancer survival was found between the women who did and did not take tamoxifen.

TABLE 5.5

Tamoxifen and Five-Year Recurrence Risks
to Women with DCIS*

Disease	No Tamoxifen	Tamoxifen
Invasive	4%	2%
Noninvasive (DCIS or LCIS)	5%	4%
Total	9%	6%

Source: Fisher et al., 1999.
*All were also treated with excision followed by radiation therapy.

The small differences in risk that were found between women who did and did not take tamoxifen may not actually be due to tamoxifen at all, since this study

- included women whose DCIS extended to the edge of the tissue. Among them were some who undoubtedly did not have all of their DCIS removed. As you learned in earlier sections, women whose DCIS is not completely removed are more likely to have a recurrence.
- did not examine all of the tissue removed to be sure that invasive breast cancer was not present along with the DCIS. Some of the women probably had undetected invasive breast cancer that was present at the start of the study. The presence of six women who devel-

oped invasive disease that spread during the relatively short time of the study supports this supposition.

Treatment Decisions

Perhaps you are wondering why a woman who is diagnosed with DCIS doesn't just have a mastectomy or radiation therapy and "be done with it." With regard to mastectomy, the most obvious reason is that few women will choose to remove their breasts unless there is evidence that it would help them. Studies to date show that if all of a woman's DCIS can be surgically removed and sufficiently clear margins are obtained, mastectomy provides no benefit. Also, mastectomy is not foolproof; invasive cancer can develop even if a woman has a mastectomy to treat her DCIS.[32]

In making a decision about radiation therapy, you may want to make use of the study results in this section, which show that when the margins are sufficiently large and clear, women who are treated with radiation have little or no reduction in their recurrence risk, suggesting that radiation treatment is more effective in treating invasive disease than DCIS. Since a breast can usually be treated only once with radiation therapy, if you should develop invasive cancer in your breast after receiving radiation therapy for DCIS, you will not be able to have more radiation treatment to that breast and will usually need a mastectomy. If, however, you are treated with surgical removal alone at the time your initial DCIS is diagnosed, radiation therapy can be used in the future if you should develop invasive disease in that breast.

Most important, remember that with proper removal of breast tissue and a thorough investigation of the tissue by a pathologist, very, very few women diagnosed with DCIS die of breast cancer. For example, in one study of 543 women, more than half of whom were followed over five years, only three died of breast cancer. *Neither radiation treatment nor tamoxifen has been found to increase a woman's already excellent survival rate after a diagnosis of DCIS.*[33] You are less likely to have a recurrence in the same breast after your diagnosis of DCIS if your treatment includes:

- Removal of all the DCIS
- Clear margins around the DCIS of at least 1 mm and preferably 1 cm
- Careful examination of all the breast tissue that is removed to be sure that invasive breast cancer is not present

- Follow-up mammography (when your breast has healed from surgery) to determine that no suspicious area remains. If such an area is present, you will want to have it removed before making treatment decisions.

This is a complex topic in which a number of important factors need to be assessed. Be sure to allow yourself time to achieve the necessary understanding, and to recover from the shock of hearing that you have an in situ "cancer." You are likely to benefit from encouragement when information seems overwhelming or confusing. Be sure you ask for it! Also, be prepared to ask until you understand. Some of the information in chapter 8 may be particularly helpful to you in navigating the medical system.

Lobular Carcinoma In Situ (LCIS)

&. Lobular carcinoma in situ (LCIS), like DCIS, lacks the ability to spread to distant parts of the body. And, like DCIS, it was identified relatively recently—in 1919. Only in 1941 was it given its current name. Because its name (which is, after all a label for particular cellular changes) includes the term carcinoma, a diagnosis of LCIS has confused and unnecessarily frightened many women over the years. To avoid confusing it with "a real cancer" or *invasive* lobular carcinoma, it has sometimes been given other names, such as lobular neoplasia.

LCIS is usually found "incidentally" when a woman has a biopsy for a breast lump or when a mammogram shows a calcification or other abnormality. That is, the LCIS is found when a biopsy is done for other reasons. It generally cannot be seen on a mammogram and does not form a lump or thickening that can be felt. For this reason, the dramatic rise in incidence that occurred with the improved mammographic detection of DCIS has not occurred for LCIS.

LCIS has been found with increased frequency in recent years, probably because more breast biopsies are being done and because pathologists are more aware of it now than they were previously. LCIS is still a rare finding, however. In a study of over 6,000 biopsies that were done after women were found to have an abnormal mammogram, LCIS was found in only about 2%.

As with DCIS, pathologists differ in the criteria they use to make a diagnosis of LCIS. What is called atypical hyperplasia by one pathologist may be called LCIS by another. And, as you might expect, the more carefully a pathologist looks and the more tissue that is examined, the more likely it is that LCIS will be found.

What is the meaning of a diagnosis of LCIS if no invasive breast cancer is found? One large study followed more than 290 women for an average of 16 years.[34] In this study women had a future breast cancer risk of about 1% a year. As a woman goes through each year without a diagnosis of breast cancer, she leaves the 1% risk for that year behind, as discussed in the section on risk over time in chapter 2. In this, and in other studies of LCIS, both breasts are about equally likely to develop invasive breast cancer in the future. That is, the risk to each breast was found to be about 0.5% a year.

The 1% a year risk of invasive breast cancer may actually be somewhat inflated, since both DCIS and LCIS were often counted as a "cancer" recurrence after a diagnosis of LCIS. For example, in one study of 99 women with LCIS, fully 30% of the "cancers" found after the LCIS diagnosis were in situ, not invasive.[35] A high proportion of the invasive and noninvasive recurrences were diagnosed years after the initial diagnosis of LCIS. In one study half the recurrences were diagnosed more than ten years after the LCIS diagnosis. In another study 38% of the recurrences were found more than twenty years after the original LCIS diagnosis.

As a result of their LCIS diagnosis, were these women more carefully followed than others, thereby increasing the chance that they would be found to have an in situ or invasive breast cancer many years later? Were these women more likely to be diagnosed with LCIS initially because they were being treated at a large medical center where investigators had a special interest in LCIS? Did a previous diagnosis of LCIS bias pathologists to interpret borderline findings in a later biopsy as LCIS or DCIS? These are possibilities in many of the studies and would, of course, influence the recurrence risks that were found.

In the future it will be possible to learn more about the natural history of LCIS since these changes are now more generally recognized by pathologists, and women are now less likely than in past years to have both breasts removed when LCIS is diagnosed. Interestingly, clear margins have *not* been shown to reduce a woman's risk of developing invasive breast cancer after a diagnosis of LCIS.

If you are considering prophylactic removal of your breasts after a

diagnosis of LCIS, be sure to read the information in chapter 10 on prophylactic mastectomy and keep the following in mind:

- The absolute risk of invasive breast cancer after a diagnosis of LCIS is
  about the same as the absolute risk after a diagnosis of atypical hyperplasia—up to 1% a year. Few women with atypical hyperplasia
  are advised to have their breasts removed. The name of the cell (LCIS)
  may well influence how future cancer risk is viewed and the treatments you are being asked to consider.
- The 1% breast cancer risk a year is shared equally by both breasts, for
  a risk of 0.5% a year per breast. As you go through each year without a diagnosis of breast cancer, you leave behind the risk associated
  with that year, as discussed in chapter 2. The risks do *not* accumulate
  over the years.
- The risk of breast cancer to all women increases with age and with
  time, so all women are at risk as they get older, not just those diagnosed with LCIS.
- Most women with LCIS never develop breast cancer.
- LCIS lacks the biological capacity to metastasize.

Some investigators believe that LCIS is a "marker" for increased breast
cancer risk but does not itself give rise to cancers in the breast because:

- The risk of cancer in future years is increased equally in both breasts.
- The types of cancers that arise after a diagnosis of LCIS vary from
  LCIS and DCIS to invasive cancers of different types.

Time and more studies will be needed to understand this issue.

Key Points to Remember

About Atypical Hyperplasia
- Benign breast disease (BBD) is an imprecise term that includes many
  different cellular and structural changes.
- Most women with BBD do not have a breast cancer risk that is higher
  than that of women in the general population.

- Women with atypical hyperplasia have a breast cancer risk of 0.5% to 1% a year.
- Women with atypical hyperplasia whose mother and/or sister were diagnosed with breast cancer have an absolute breast cancer risk that is no greater than their absolute risk due to family history alone.

About DCIS

- DCIS lacks the biological capacity to metastasize.
- In making a treatment decision about DCIS be sure to learn:
  - The type of DCIS
  - The size of the DCIS
  - The size of the margin of clear tissue around the DCIS
  - Whether any suspicious calcifications that were seen on the mammogram before surgery remain after surgery. If any do, most experts advise that they be removed.
- In one study women with clear surgical margins of 1 cm or greater around their DCIS had at most an invasive breast cancer risk of about 1% a year—about the same risk as a woman diagnosed with atypical hyperplasia. With larger clear margins the recurrence risks are smaller, which means that cosmetic considerations need to be balanced with the clear benefits of a wide margin.
- Women with DCIS who are treated with radiation therapy and/or tamoxifen do not live longer than women treated with surgical removal of the DCIS alone. Both groups have an excellent prognosis, since DCIS does not metastasize.
- The group of women with a DCIS diagnosis most likely to benefit from radiation treatment is not now known.
- Radiation treatment does *not* decrease a woman's recurrence risk after a diagnosis of DCIS if the margins around the DCIS are not clear.

About LCIS

- LCIS lacks the biological capacity to metastasize.
- The absolute risk of invasive breast cancer after a diagnosis of LCIS is about 1% a year—about the same risk as a woman diagnosed with atypical hyperplasia, which ranges from 0.5% to 1% a year.

Hormone Replacement Therapy (HRT) and Breast Cancer Risk

> My business is to teach my aspirations to conform themselves
> to fact, not to try and make facts harmonize with my aspira-
> tions.
>
> Thomas Henry Huxley, 1860, cited in Taubes, 1998[1]

Many people assume that a woman who takes hormones at menopause substantially increases her breast cancer risk. In this chapter I review many of the major studies in this area. As you will see, in most studies women who take hormones at menopause do not have a higher breast cancer risk than nonusers. In those few instances in which a statistically significant increase in risk is present, it represents quite a small risk in absolute terms.

You may also have heard that we need more studies about the effects of hormone replacement therapy (HRT) on a woman's breast cancer risk before the jury is in. However, as I show in this chapter, the large number of studies investigating this issue from a variety of perspectives has created such a wide and solid information base, that it will be very difficult for future studies to overturn the current body of evidence.

Why, then, do we hear so much about a woman's risk of breast cancer if she takes HRT? At least some of the concern appears to be based on a reliance on relative risk (which is a comparison of one group's risk to that of another) and a failure to assess study results in a consistent and appropriate manner. For example, as Gardner and Altman point out in their book, *Statistics with Confidence*: "There is a tendency to equate statistical significance with medical importance or biological relevance."[2] They suggest a different approach: "In medical studies investigators should usually be interested in determining the *size of difference* [italics are mine] of a measured outcome between groups, rather than a simple indication of whether or not it is statistically significant."

To assist *you* in evaluating study results, I begin this chapter with a brief description of epidemiology (the study of diseases in populations) and five criteria used to evaluate epidemiologic studies. As you will see, the criteria are straightforward, based on common sense, and easy to apply. When you use them, you will be less likely to be misled by study results, and the relevance of these results to your situation will be clearer.

Epidemiologic Studies

When most of us think of a scientific study, we think of one involving cause and effect. In this type of study an antibiotic (cause) might be added to a cell culture to see if it produces a change (effect) in the cells. In contrast, epidemiologic studies are not studies of cause and effect. Most, like the studies discussed in this chapter, are studies of association, and compare the rates of disease in a group that is exposed to an agent (such as HRT) with the disease rate in a group not exposed to the agent. Studies of this type cannot determine whether HRT *causes* breast cancer or promotes its growth, but instead provide information about associations between HRT use and breast cancer. When an association (either an increase or a decrease in risk) is present, *further assessment is needed to determine whether the association is or is not causal*. Without this assessment, misunderstandings about the importance of a study's result can occur. In this section I will show you how commonsense this assessment is.

In epidemiology, the gold standard is the "randomized prospective study" in which, for example, a large group of women from similar backgrounds and having similar breast cancer risks would be randomly assigned to either take or not take HRT, then followed for some years to see what differences in breast cancer risk occurred between the two groups. With large enough groups, other factors that might influence breast cancer risk would probably be evenly distributed between the two groups, so any difference in breast cancer rates would likely be due to HRT and not to these other factors. Randomized studies can be costly, and it can take years before results are obtained—twenty years, for example. For these and other reasons randomized studies are not conducted nearly as often as observational studies.

The studies about breast cancer risk and HRT use that you've heard about and that I'll discuss in this chapter are observational. In an observational study, the rate of breast cancer in a group of women who took HRT might be compared to the breast cancer rate in a group that did not take hormones. In such a study, if a difference in breast cancer rate between the two groups is found, it might be due to HRT use. It could also occur if the two groups were composed of women who had different breast cancer risks that were unrelated to HRT use. Since many breast cancer risks are currently unknown, a difference in risk between groups due to other factors can be a real possibility, no matter how carefully groups are matched according to known risks.

Unknown factors can influence results in even the most carefully constructed study. For example, if we didn't know that the products of cigarette smoking increase lung cancer risk, we could be misled by finding that a group of women with matches in their pockets had a higher risk of lung cancer than a group that had no matches in their pockets. This could easily lead to more and more studies of brands of matches, right-pocket versus left-pocket matches, etc. No matter how elegantly structured these studies were, no matter how sophisticated the statistical analysis of the results, the unwary might conclude that matches increase lung cancer risk. Many of the factors that increase breast cancer risk are not yet known, so investigators have no way to devise observational studies to exclude their effects in HRT (or other) studies.

Assessment Criteria

To avoid being misled by associations that are not causative (like the matches and lung cancer) and to determine the likelihood that a particular agent, such as HRT, is causative, epidemiologists use the following five criteria:

1. Timing. Did exposure to the agent occur before the onset of disease? Most breast cancers grow for seven to ten years before they are detected. Therefore, in a study of women who use HRT for less than seven to ten years, most or all of the breast cancers found are likely to have been present *before* HRT use began. HRT is therefore unlikely to be a causative agent for breast cancers that are found in the first seven to ten years after a woman starts using HRT. I discuss the likelihood that HRT use might *promote* the growth of breast cancer cells that are already present in this chapter's section, "HRT Use and Developing Cancers."

2. *Similar findings in many studies.* Any one observational study is subject to influences from known and unknown factors, so information is more accurate when the same result is found in a number of studies. The link between lung cancer and cigarette smoking, for example, is not confined to one study but is found in many.

3. *A risk that increases as dose increases and that decreases when the dose is decreased or the agent is removed.*

4. *Statistically significant differences.* Tests of statistical significance are used to determine whether the difference between the risks in two groups is larger than you would expect if you were to select other similar groups from the same overall large population. In other words, the test is done to determine whether the difference in risk is likely to be due to the way the two groups were chosen for study or is likely to be due to the agent being studied. If a difference in risk is *not* statistically significant, the way the groups were chosen probably accounts for the difference in risk between the two groups. If the difference *is* statistically significant, the agent being studied, such as HRT, *may* account for the difference.

A significance test commonly used in medical studies has what is called a "95% confidence interval." In such a case there is a 5% chance that a significant difference will be obtained as a result of the way the groups are selected from the overall population, not to any "real" difference in risk. Such a statistical difference can mislead you into thinking that the difference in risk is greater than you would expect, when it actually is not. Therefore, *no one statistical difference is conclusive.* The other main point is that statistically significant differences can be large or small, important or unimportant. The test addresses only the likelihood that you would continue to obtain as large or larger differences in risk if you continued to select groups from the same population pool—such as women who take hormones and women in their neighborhood who do not.

5. The presence of a large effect. Observational study results may be influenced by differences between study groups that are unrelated to the agent being studied. That is, an association may be found that is not causal, *even if the difference in risk is statistically significant.* In my example about matches in pockets an association was found between the matches and lung cancer risk. However, it was not causal since the matches did not cause the lung cancer.

To avoid being misled by associations that are not causal, epidemiologists look for a difference in risk that is statistically significant *and* is threefold or greater. When the relative risk is less than three, other factors, they point out, not the agent being studied, could explain the results. For example, if a relative risk is fourfold and is statistically significant, it is more likely that the agent being studied is responsible for the difference found than if the relative risk is 1.5.

One way you can avoid being misled by unknown factors that cannot be taken into account in a study's design is to be cautious about accepting the usefulness of studies that report small differences in risk. As one well-known scientist bluntly said in the journal *Science*, if the relative risk found "isn't at least three or four, forget it."[3]

As you read the descriptions of the studies on HRT that follow, you might refer to this list, which epidemiologists themselves have long used as guidelines. You will see that when you apply these criteria, HRT does not appear to be a causative agent or one that promotes the growth of breast cancers to any appreciable extent.

Comparison Risks

The results of epidemiologic studies are reported as comparison risks (called "relative risks" or "odds ratio" in scientific studies). With both relative risks and odds ratios, the risk to a group without the disease or without the risk factor being studied is assigned a baseline risk of 1.0. Rates in the other group (with the disease or with the risk factor) are then compared to the baseline rate. In this book I refer to both relative risks and odds ratios as relative risks.

A relative risk of 1.0 means, for example, that during the time covered by the study a group taking HRT and a group not taking HRT developed equivalent rates of breast cancer. A relative risk of less than one, such as 0.8, means that the group taking HRT had a lower breast cancer rate than the group not taking HRT. A relative risk greater than 1.0, such as 1.5, means that the group taking HRT had 1.5 times as much breast cancer as the group that didn't take HRT. A relative risk of 0.8 is also called a 20% reduction in risk, while 1.5 is called a 50% increase in risk. I've shown this method of reporting risks in figure 10.

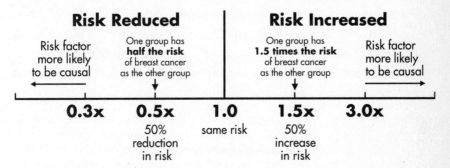

Figure 10. Relative Risk and Likelihood That Risk Factor Is Causal

Most studies in this area compare breast cancer rates in women who use HRT with those of nonusers. As a group, non-hormone users generally have fewer mammograms and breast examinations than women who take hormones, since most physicians will not prescribe HRT unless a woman has a yearly physical breast examination and a mammogram. Obviously, in a group of women having more mammograms and breast examinations, breast cancers are more likely to be found than in a group having fewer or none. As you will see, even with this built-in bias, in most studies women who use HRT *do not have a statistically significant increase in breast cancer risk*. In the few instances in which statistical significance is present, the relative risks are less than three. More important, the absolute risks are small.

Estrogen Dose

⌔ If HRT is a causative agent, or a causative agent to any extent that can be measured, we would expect that women who used a higher hormone dose would have a greater breast cancer risk than those who used less or who used none. After all, if most of us eat more, we gain weight; when we reduce the amount of food we eat, we tend to lose weight. The more cigarettes a person smokes, the higher the risk of lung cancer.

In HRT studies, women who take a higher dose of estrogen do not have a greater risk of breast cancer than those who take less or who take none. For example, in a large study of nurses, women who used from 0.3 milligrams (mg) to more than 1.25 mg of estrogen a day did not have a higher risk than nonusers.[4] Most hormone users take at least 0.625 mg of estrogen a day to protect their bones and heart, but some use 2.0 mg or more, since metabolism rates differ. Several other studies also find that women who take a higher dose of HRT are not at greater breast cancer risk than those who take lower doses or do not use hormones at all.

Years of Estrogen Use

◈ But what about use over time? Does a woman's breast cancer risk increase with the number of years she has been taking hormones? After all you have read and heard, you may be surprised to learn that in many studies women who use HRT for ten or even up to twenty years do *not* have a higher breast cancer risk than women who never use hormones. (The type of hormone women use at menopause has changed over the years.) Most long-term users took estrogen only, and of a particular type called Premarin. In recent years far more choices and hormone combinations have become available. I discuss some of them below in "Estrogen and Progesterone Use."

In one particularly well-designed study, women who used hormones for up to twenty years had no statistically significant increase in breast cancer risk compared to nonusers.[5] I've listed these results in table 6.1. The left column shows years of hormone use from less than five years all the way up to twenty or more years. The next column shows the relative risk found in each of the time intervals. For example, with less than five years' use women who took HRT had 0.8 times the risk of nonusers—a slightly lower risk. From five to nine years the risk was 1.1 times that of nonusers— a slightly higher risk.

None of the relative risks in this study is statistically significant, so the difference in risk between users and nonusers is not likely to be due to hor-

TABLE 6.1

Years of HRT Use and Breast Cancer Risk (Study 1)

Years HRT Used	Relative Risk*
Less than 5	0.8
5–9	1.1
10–14	1.3
15–10	1.2
20 or more	1.5

Source: Briton et al., 1986.
*None is statistically significant; all are less than threefold, so it is likely that factors other than HRT are responsible for the differences in risk.

mone use. The 1.5 relative risk after twenty years is higher than that for any of the other time periods. Notice, however, that it is not statistically significant and does not approach the three- or fourfold difference that is needed to rule out the effects of unknown factors. In many studies the group followed for the longest time has smaller numbers of women in it than the others. With smaller numbers, fluctuations in risk are more likely, so risks in the last category may differ from those in preceding years that have larger numbers.

Women in another study who used HRT for fifteen or more years did not have a statistically significant increase in breast cancer risk compared to nonusers.[6] The results of this study are shown in table 6.2. Note that all the way up to fourteen years women who used hormones had a 0.9- to 0.7-fold *decrease* in relative risk compared to nonusers. The differences were not statistically significant and were not large. Therefore, one cannot reasonably conclude from this study that women who use HRT have a *decreased* breast cancer risk. The last category (women who used hormones for 15 or more years) contained fewer women than other categories and also showed a greater difference than the others. Again, this difference was not statistically significant and was far less than the three- or fourfold increase discussed earlier. This difference is therefore not likely to be due to HRT use.

TABLE 6.2

Years of HRT Use and Breast Cancer Risk (Study 2)

Years HRT Used	Relative Risk*
Less than 1	0.9
1–4	0.7
5–9	0.9
10–14	0.7
15 or more	1.5

Source: Palmer et al., 1991.
*None is statistically significant; all are less than threefold, so it is likely that factors other than HRT are responsible for the differences in risk.

A third study investigated the breast cancer risk to women who used HRT for 20 or more years.[7] In this study also, women's risks of breast cancer did not increase as they used hormones for longer time periods. I've shown the results of this study in table 6.3. As you can see, most of the relative risks hover around 1.0 and are not statistically significant. From eight to eleven years, hormone users actually had a *decrease* in the relative risk of breast cancer that *was* statistically significant. However, there were fewer than 50 women in one of the two comparison groups, so the difference in breast cancer risk may be due to the small numbers studied and not to HRT use, even though statistical significance was present. Several studies would need to find a statistically significant decrease in relative risk for this length of hormone use before it would be reasonable to conclude that the decrease in risk was due to HRT use.

At this point you may be wondering why you have heard so much about an increase in breast cancer risk with increasing years of HRT use if it isn't present in most studies. I think the (erroneous) focus has been on very small increases in relative risk without an appreciation of how small these risks actually are in absolute risk terms. For example, if a 1.3 relative risk is reported as a 30% increase, that sounds large, even though, as you will see in the next section, the absolute risk is less than 1 in 100 women over ten years.

TABLE 6.5

Breast Cancer Risk to Women Currently Using HRT
Compared to Never Users

Years Used	Relative Risk
Up to 2	1.1
2–4	1.2
5–9	1.5*
10 or more	1.5*

Source: Colditz et al., 1995.
*Significant.

multiple groups to study from the overall population. It's like a 5% error rate.

The other important point to appreciate is that comparison of breast cancer rates in two groups is imprecise. As you may remember from the criteria listed at the beginning of this chapter, when relative risks are three or less, even if they are statistically significant, the difference may be due to "background noise" and not to the agent being studied. According to an article in the journal *Science*, "Epidemiology Faces Its Limits," "Many epidemiologists interviewed by *Science* say that risk-factor epidemiology is increasingly straying beyond the limits of the possible no matter how carefully the studies are done." It also reported, "Many epidemiologists concede that their studies are so plagued with biases, uncertainties, and methodological weaknesses that they may be inherently incapable of accurately discerning such weak [30% or 1.3] associations."[10]

But what if the 1.5 relative risk with ten or more years of hormone use that was present in the nurses study *is* actually due to HRT use and not to undetected differences in risk between the study groups, to differences in numbers of mammograms, or to cancers that were present before hormone use started? You may remember that most breast cancers grow seven to ten years before they are detected, so cancers found in the first five to ten years after a woman takes HRT are likely to have been present when her hormone use started.

When this study was published, the average woman's breast cancer risk was 5% from age 50 to 70. A 1.5 relative risk would mean, in approximate absolute risk terms, a 7.5% risk (the relative risk of 1.5 × the 5% average woman's risk from 50 to 70 = 7.5%). That is, with HRT use one would find a 7.5% absolute risk—an increase of 2.5% *spread over twenty years*. A 2.5% risk divided by twenty years is only 0.125%—less than one-eighth of one percent a year. Breast cancer risk goes up with age, so the 0.125% is not spread evenly across the twenty years. However, this gives you a general idea of how small such a risk would be each year. Differences of this size are probably too small for observational studies to detect with any reliability—what the *Science* article called "epidemiology stretched to its limits or beyond."

Another, more sophisticated, approach used original data from nearly all of the major studies on length of HRT use that were published up to 1997.[11] The authors included in their calculations the following assumptions:

- A woman starts HRT use at age 50.
- A woman uses HRT for ten years.
- HRT use increases breast cancer risk by 30% to 50% (1.3 to 1.5 in relative risk terms).

With these assumptions, they calculated that a relative risk of 1.3 to 1.5 was equivalent to an absolute risk of only 0.6 additional cases of breast cancer *per 100 women* up to age 70. That's right, with a 30% to 50% increase in risk, less than one additional case of breast cancer would occur in 100 women from age 50 all the way up to age 70 if they all used HRT from age 50 to 60. This is another example of how misleading risk statements can be when they are couched in terms of a percentage increase or decrease, and underscores the usefulness of absolute risks in making individual decisions.

In summary, most studies find no statistically significant increase in relative risk of breast cancer when women use HRT for fifteen or even twenty years. In one study that did find a statistically significant increase in relative risk after five years of hormone use, the increase may have been at least partially due to more frequent mammograms among HRT users than nonusers. The 1.5 relative risk in this study might also be due to factors other than HRT use since it is less than the three- to four-fold increase discussed earlier. However, even if the 1.5 relative risk in this study *is* due to HRT use, this increase means that less than one additional case of breast cancer would be found in 100 women from age 50 up to age 70 if they used hormones for ten years.

Estrogen and Progesterone Use

Until the 1980s most women who took hormones at menopause used estrogen only. When it became apparent that the use of estrogen alone increased a woman's risk of endometrial (uterine) cancer, women began taking both estrogen and a modified type of progesterone. Progesterone is a hormone that prepares a woman's uterus for fertilization. Until recently only modified forms of progesterone were used. Increasingly, women who use progesterone take a natural, unmodified type.

A number of studies have investigated the risk of breast cancer to women who take both estrogen and progesterone and found they had no increase in risk of breast cancer.[12] A more recent study raised concerns about risks associated with estrogen and progesterone when it reported that women who took estrogen and a synthetic progesterone (called progestin) had an 8% increase in breast cancer risk each year.[13] Those who were thin had a 12% increase each year.

Let's take a look at what this 12% increase actually means. Because it is 12% greater than a very small risk, in absolute terms, it turns out that *two thousand women* would need to take estrogen and a modified progesterone for one year before even one additional breast cancer would be detected. I use the term "detected" here instead of "caused," since this study has not shown cause. Most of the increases in risk that were statistically significant occurred in the first four years of hormone use, so all or most of the additional cancers were probably present when the women started using hormones. In this study the breast cancers that were found in hormone users were not larger or more aggressive than those in nonusers, suggesting that hormone use did not accelerate tumor growth.

As a whole, then, studies on risk of breast cancer to women who take estrogen and a progesterone (largely modified progesterone to date) do not find an increased breast cancer risk or find one that is quite small. The use of estrogen and progesterone is relatively recent, so these studies have smaller numbers of women and shorter follow-up times than studies of women who used estrogen alone. Increasingly, women are using a natural progesterone, so more studies are needed as this use grows.

Family History of Breast Cancer

There are now at least six studies of risk to women who have one or more close relative with breast cancer and who use HRT.[14] In each study, women who used HRT did not have an increased breast cancer risk compared to nonusers with similar family histories.

Occasionally a colleague will show me a reference to a study that reports an increased breast cancer risk to users of HRT who have a family history of breast cancer. When I investigate the studies themselves, I find that they include fewer than 50 (sometimes fewer than 20) women with breast cancer—not enough to produce reliable results.

Benign Breast Disease

Some women assume that if they were diagnosed with benign breast disease they would be foolish to take hormones at menopause. The evidence does not support their concern. In a number of studies women with various types of benign breast disease who take HRT do not have an increased breast cancer risk. Even women with atypical hyperplasia, a type of benign breast disease that is itself associated with an increased breast cancer risk, do not further increase their risk by taking hormones. (For more about atypical hyperplasia, see chapter 5.) In the few studies that *do* find an increase in breast cancer risk to women with benign breast disease who use HRT, each has fewer than 50 women with breast cancer in any one group—not enough to generate meaningful absolute risks. Also, in those few instances when a statistically significant increase in breast cancer risk is found, the relative risk is less than the three- to fourfold increase that is needed to rule out noise in the system.

HRT Use and Developing Cancers

What if a woman has a cancer cell (or more) in her breast when she starts taking HRT? Is this like pouring gasoline on a fire? Let's see what we can learn from a number of recent studies of women who *were* using HRT when their breast cancer was diagnosed. Remember, the cells that make up a breast cancer grow seven to ten years in a woman's breast before they are usually detected. Therefore, many women whose breast cancers were diagnosed while they were taking HRT actually had breast cancer before their hormone use began and used HRT for years while a cancer was in their breasts. These women unknowingly contributed to a natural, unplanned study of the effects of HRT on a growing breast cancer. What were their cancers like? What happened to these women?

The results are again most encouraging and reassuring. In study after study, women who were taking HRT at the time of their breast cancer diagnosis are found to live *at least as long* as women who were not taking hormones at the time of their diagnosis.[15] The results of one study are shown in figure 11.[16] The arrow at the bottom of the graph indicates the point at which the women in this study were diagnosed with breast cancer. Survival is shown at the side in percentages, with longer survival toward the top of the graph. As you can see, the women who were taking HRT at the time of their breast cancer diagnosis were more likely to be alive at the end of fifteen years than those who had never used HRT.

When I first saw these results, I wondered if the women who used HRT lived longer because they saw their doctor more regularly or had more frequent mammograms than women who were not taking hormones. More frequent medical attention would then give HRT users a better chance of finding their breast cancers at smaller sizes, which would increase their survival rates.

Several studies have investigated this issue. In some studies women who were taking HRT did have smaller breast cancers than those who were not taking HRT when their breast cancer was diagnosed. In other studies both groups of women had their breast cancers diagnosed at similar sizes. However, even among women whose breast cancers were diagnosed at large sizes, or who had cancer in the lymph nodes under the arm, those who were using HRT when their breast cancer was diagnosed had a survival

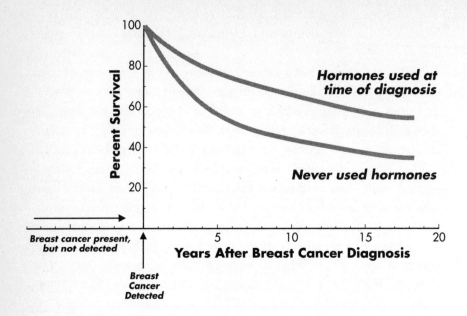

Figure 11. Survival of Women Who Were Diagnosed
with Breast Cancer While Using HRT
Source: Adapted from Strickland et al., 1992.

rate *as good as or better* than that of women who were not taking hormones. Women taking hormones do NOT have more aggressive or more
rapidly dividing tumors (as defined by the numbers of dividing cells and
cell appearance) than nonusers.[17] If HRT use stimulated tumor growth
you would expect that the cancers in women who were using HRT would
be dividing more rapidly than breast cancers in nonusers. This is not
the case.

As a group, then, studies find that women who are using HRT while a
breast cancer is present in their breasts have:

- Breast cancers that are no larger than those present in women who
  are nonusers. This suggests that HRT use does not stimulate breast
  cancer growth. If it did, women taking HRT would have, on average,
  larger breast cancers than nonusers.
- Breast cancers that are not more rapidly growing than cancers found

in nonusers. This suggests that HRT use does not stimulate the growth of breast cancer to any measurable extent.

• At least as good a prognosis as non-hormone users, regardless of breast cancer size. This suggests that HRT use at menopause does not stimulate cancer growth and is not dangerous, even if a woman should, unknown to her, have a cancer cell or cells in her breast.

Hormone Use and Mortality

Almost all studies show an *improved* life expectancy for HRT users compared to women who are not taking hormones. For example, in a large nurses study, women taking hormones at menopause had a 0.6 relative risk of dying of *all* causes compared to women who never used hormones.[18] As you can see in table 6.6, this decrease in overall death rate was statistically significant. Hormone users were half as likely to die of heart disease as non-hormone users. Risk of death due to all cancers was somewhat decreased and was statistically significant.

TABLE 6.6

Risk of Death to Women
Using HRT Compared to Nonusers

Cause of Death	Relative Risk
All Deaths	0.6*
Heart Disease	0.5*
Stroke	0.7
All Cancers	0.7*
Breast Cancer	0.8

Source: Grodstein et al., 1997.
*Significant.

Because none of the relative risks was reduced to the 0.4 or 0.3 level, these differences in risk between users and nonusers, even though statistically significant, may be due to differences in lifestyle factors, and not to HRT use. This study's results, therefore, do not provide definitive evidence that HRT use *decreases* a woman's risk of death. They do show, however, that hormone users were no more likely to die of breast cancer than nonusers of hormones. The 0.8 relative risk of breast cancer is not statistically significant, which means that the slight reduction in risk of death to HRT users is likely to be due to other causes, not HRT use.

A number of other studies find that women using HRT have either a decreased breast cancer death rate or no increase in death rate, compared to women who are not using hormones. Table 6.7 shows the results of one of these studies in which the breast cancer death rate in women who used HRT for eleven or more years was compared to that of non-hormone users.[19] Notice that some of the decreases in death rates for hormone users are statistically significant. That is, women taking HRT are less likely to die of breast cancer than nonusers. Here the relative risks are not small enough to rule out the effects of factors other than HRT use. This study, like others, does show that women who take HRT live at least as long as those who are nonusers.

TABLE 6.7

Years of HRT Use and Risk of Death Due to Breast Cancer

Years Used	Relative Risk
Never	1.0 (comparison group)
Less than 1	0.9
2–5	0.8*
6–10	0.8*
11 or more	0.9

Source: Willis et al., 1996.
*Significant.

Women who have a mother or sister with breast cancer and who use HRT are not more likely to die of breast cancer than nonusers with similar family histories.[20] As a group, then, studies find that women who use HRT are not more likely to die of breast or other cancers than are nonusers.

Use after a Breast Cancer Diagnosis

The use of HRT after a woman has been diagnosed with breast cancer is controversial. Some say that not enough studies have been done to warrant its use in this circumstance. What do the studies show? To date, relatively few women who take HRT after their breast cancer diagnosis have been studied. In the studies that are available, HRT users either have a better prognosis or a prognosis that is as good as that of women who do not take hormones. For example, in one study of 90 women who used hormones for up to twelve years after a breast cancer diagnosis, 7% had a recurrence, compared to a 17% recurrence in women who did not use hormones.[21] None of the hormone users died, but 6% of the nonusers did.

Other studies, with smaller numbers, have similar findings.[22] That is, they find no increase in risk of breast cancer recurrence or death to women who take hormones after a breast cancer diagnosis, compared to those who do not. A 1999 prospective study of 39 women who took HRT and 280 who did not, all of whom had been diagnosed with breast cancer, reported that at the end of nine and a half years, only one of the hormone users and fourteen of the nonusers had developed a recurrence.[23] These studies suggest that use of HRT after a breast cancer diagnosis does not worsen a woman's prognosis. More studies will be needed in this area before these results can be considered conclusive, of course.

I increasingly hear about women who are taking HRT after their breast cancer diagnosis. This treatment is not the standard of care in medical communities, so if a woman decides to take hormones after her diagnosis she must strongly push for it. Often this means looking around for a doctor who is willing to prescribe in such cases.

HRT and Heart Disease

One of my patients, Alice, told me she was not concerned about her risk of heart disease after menopause, since heart disease does not run in her family. I explained that most heart disease in 55- to 74-year old women is not due to strong hereditary factors, but appears to result from the aging process itself. Before age 50, women are unlikely to die of heart disease, but after this time the rate increases rapidly. In 1999 over 100,000 women between the ages of 55 and 74 were estimated to die of heart diseases, compared to an estimated 20,000 or fewer deaths due to breast cancer.[24] Women aged 50 to 54 are about as likely to die of heart disease as breast cancer.[25] However, by age 60, breast cancer accounts for a little over 10% of all deaths, and heart disease about 20%. At age 70, breast cancer deaths constitute less than 10% of all deaths, while nearly 30% of the deaths are due to heart disease. These figures demonstrate how steeply heart disease deaths among women rise after age 55.

In a number of studies women taking hormones were about half as likely to die of heart disease compared to women not taking hormones.[26] Estrogen may help prevent heart disease by reducing several factors that increase risk—decreasing cholesterol levels, for example.

In the last year several media reports have cast doubt on the effectiveness of HRT in protecting women from heart disease and have suggested that HRT use may even increase this risk. The reports generally failed to make it plain that in these studies, all of the women already had diagnosed heart disease. And the actual number of women experiencing a heart-related problem during the study was very small. In one case, the results were so preliminary that the investigators themselves cautioned that they could be due to chance. In any event, these studies do not provide information about the risk of heart disease to women *without* a diagnosis of heart disease who take HRT.

But what about women with diagnosed heart disease? Should they be taking hormones at menopause? Here the story becomes complex. In the best known study, which was a randomized prospective study (see page 111 for a discussion about this type of study), over 1,300 women took HRT and 1,300 did not.[27] At the end of four years, 5.5% of the HRT users and 4.5% of the nonusers had died of heart disease. The difference was not statistically significant. However, in the first year of the study HRT users did have a higher risk that was statistically significant. Because the study was of the randomized prospective type its results caused some to conclude that HRT increases a woman's risk of heart disease.

A closer look at this study, however, reveals that factors other than study design may account for the difference in results found between it and previous studies. One possibility is that the types of hormones used may have influenced the results. In this study women took both estrogen and a modified progesterone every day. Many physicians do not prescribe modified progesterone to women with heart disease because they are concerned about its possible harmful effects to women in this group. Instead, they prescribe a *natural* progesterone which has beneficial effects on cholesterol that can help to reduce a woman's risk of heart disease. So, one possibility for the increase in risk could be the type of progesterone that was used.

Another possibility is that the increase in risk arose from the way in which women took these hormones—both hormones were taken every day of the month. Some physicians tell me that they are concerned about exposing women with known heart disease to any type of progesterone every day. Instead they suggest that women with heart disease take estrogen all month, but progesterone for only about ten or twelve days a month. In the earlier studies that found a significant decrease in heart disease risk, the women were taking estrogen only, so the difference in the hormones taken is a plausible reason for the difference found.

Another factor that might account for the increased risk of heart disease among hormone users in the randomized study may be that a number of the women who were using hormones stopped taking them suddenly. They did so largely due to unpleasant side effects that may have been brought about by taking the total dose immediately, instead of starting slowly and building up.[28] The increase in heart disease risk to this group might therefore have been due to a sudden withdrawal of hormones that could lead to a spasm in these women's already damaged arteries. You can see that more studies are needed to put the results of this study in perspective.

This section is by no means intended to be a comprehensive review of the many studies on heart disease risk and HRT use. I mention some of the studies and controversies here so you can see what a complex area this is.

Many factors, including the presence or absence of heart disease, types of hormones a woman uses, and the schedule she uses to take them all need to be addressed. In these studies, as in studies on HRT and breast cancer risk, care must be taken in interpreting the results. Clearly more studies are needed in this area—studies of women with and without heart disease and studies of women taking different types of hormones on differing schedules.

Who Should Use HRT?

As a group, a considerable number of epidemiologic studies do not provide evidence of an appreciable increase in breast cancer risk to women who use hormones at menopause. Some studies find a decrease in risk of heart disease while others, including a large prospective study of women who already had heart disease and who took estrogen and a modified progesterones, do not.

Some studies report a reduced risk of Alzheimer's disease and colon cancer to women who take HRT. This might be due to estrogen's ability to convert oxygen free radicals to less harmful products. (Oxygen free radicals are breakdown products of the foods that we eat and are formed during the natural workings of our bodies. They are thought to damage the cell's genes, which in turn can increase cancer risk.) By contributing to damage to blood vessel walls, oxygen free radicals are thought to increase the risk of heart disease. Estrogen has a great capacity to neutralize oxygen free radicals and so is thought to decrease or eliminate the damage they cause. A number of studies find that women who take hormones are less likely to develop osteoporosis, a thinning of the bones that can lead to broken bones and a decrease in both quality and quantity of life.

What do all of these study results, some of them preliminary, mean to you? Should you take hormones? With HRT, as with eyeglasses or inoculations, it is only common sense to have a reason for using it. Some women go through menopause with no problems or discomforts and have little or no reason to be concerned about their risks of bone fracture, heart disease, or some of the other diseases mentioned above. Others suffer great discomfort during the menopausal years and after. Symptoms and concerns differ, which means that no one approach is right for all.

My aim in this chapter has been to provide information that will be useful to you in making up your mind if you, like many of the women I see, would "go on HRT in a second" or if you would like to take a higher hormone dose to feel comfortable, but have been afraid that by doing so you will increase your breast cancer risk to an appreciable extent. As you can see from the evidence presented, HRT either does not increase breast cancer risk or does so to an extent that influences an individual woman's risk to a very minor extent.

If you decide to take HRT, be sure to consult with a physician who has experience in prescribing hormones. This is a rapidly growing subspecialty. In Appendix B I have listed a national center that can help you to find such physicians. Also, be aware that you have a number of different hormone options, some of which may be better suited to you than others. Be sure to communicate with your doctor about how you are feeling, and any past medical problems.

Key Points to Remember

- To evaluate the likelihood that an agent, such as HRT, is causative, epidemiologic studies are evaluated as a group. Important criteria used to evaluate these study results include:
    - Exposure to an agent such as HRT before onset of disease
    - Similar findings in several studies
    - An effect that increases with dose and decreases when use stops
    - Statistically significant differences in risk
    - The presence of a strong effect, such as a relative risk of three or greater.
- Most studies find no increased risk of breast cancer to women who use HRT when:
    - The dose of HRT increases
    - HRT is used for up to twenty years
    - A woman has a close relative with breast cancer
    - A woman has benign breast disease.
- Women who are diagnosed with breast cancer while taking HRT have a prognosis at least as good as women who are not using hormones at the time of their diagnosis.

SEVEN

Some of Those "Other" Risks:
Reproductive History, Diet,
Alcohol, and the Pill

We read and hear a great deal about the effects of a woman's reproductive history, diet, alcohol consumption, and oral contraceptives on her breast cancer risk—so much, in fact, that you may be surprised to learn that these factors influence an individual woman's breast cancer risks little, if at all. Why, then, are they discussed so often? I am not sure, but I have several thoughts. One is that plausible theories to explain how these factors might influence risk have been discussed for years, so the discussion has become habitual. The other is that by having information about something, even small differences, scientists and the public can feel that some progress is being made in learning about the causes of breast cancer. As you will see, the differences in absolute numbers are so small, when they are present at all, that the amount of attention these factors receive is completely out of proportion to their significance.

The information we have about risk of breast cancer and the factors mentioned above is largely derived from epidemiologic studies, not studies of cause and effect. As I discussed in chapter 6, an increase in risk that is found in an epidemiologic study needs to be evaluated to determine the likelihood that the agent being studied is actually responsible for the effect that is present. An agent is more likely to be the cause of a disease when all of the following criteria are met:

- Exposure to the agent occurs before the onset of disease.
- Similar findings are obtained in many studies.

- Risk increases when the dose increases, and decreases when the dose decreases or is removed.
- Statistically significant differences are present.
- The relative risk is threefold or greater.

These guidelines, which are discussed in chapter 6, will help you to evaluate the study results presented in this chapter.

Reproductive History—How Much Does It Really Matter?

Even though reproductive history is generally listed as a "minor risk factor" for breast cancer, women often tell me, "I know my breast cancer risk must be high since I haven't had a child." As I review their family history, they may say, "I was only eleven when I started my periods, so I guess that puts me in a high-risk category." When I hear these comments, I can hardly wait to show a woman that the increase in risk is not nearly as solidly established or as large as she may believe. In this section I will show you, too.

Here I review studies about the effects of a wide range of reproductive history factors on an individual's breast cancer risk:

- Age when she started menstruation (also called "age at menarche")
- Age when her first child was born—or if she has not given birth to a child
- Fertility drug use
- Breast-feeding
- Age at menopause

Age When Menstruation Begins

You may have heard that women who start their periods when they are older have a lower breast cancer risk than those who start at younger ages. Let's take a look at what the study results show in this regard. In a report of four separate studies, breast cancer risks to women who started their periods at 12, 13, and so on up to age 17 and older were compared to the risks to women whose periods started at age 11 and younger. In two of the four studies, a significant reduction in risk was found—but only when women who started their periods at 17 and older were compared to women whose periods began at 11 and younger. And both of these groups represented a small percentage of the population. In these two instances the relative risks were less than threefold. *None* of the other comparisons for any of the other ages *resulted in differences that were significant in any of the four studies.*[1]

You may remember from chapter 6 that comparisons of risks between two groups are reported as "relative risks" or "odds ratios" and that I am calling both relative risks. When the groups being studied have the same risk, it is written as 1.0. When the group having the factor under investigation has a higher risk, it is written as a number greater than one, such as 1.3. When the risk is lower, it is written as less than one, such as 0.8. When a relative risk is less than threefold, factors other than the agent being studied may well be responsible for the difference in risk that is present.

In other studies also, significant differences are rarely present, and when they are, the differences are generally found between small groups at either end of the spectrum, the relative risk is less than threefold, and the absolute risks are small. As a group, these studies do not provide evidence that a woman's age at the time of her first period has a consequential effect on her breast cancer risk.

Age at First Period and Family History of Breast Cancer

In several studies, women who had a mother or sister with breast cancer and whose periods started at older ages did not have statistically significant decreases in breast cancer risk compared to those with similar family histories whose periods began at 12 and younger.[2] In another study, women who had at least two close relatives with breast cancer and who were 13 or older when they started their first periods had a lower breast cancer risk than those who were 12 and younger when their first periods began.[3] However, in this study the groups that are compared contain wide ranges in age. Such results therefore apply to the group and not to any one age in the group. The available evidence to date suggests that there is little or no interaction in risk between family history of breast cancer and the age when a woman starts menstruation.

Childbirth

You may have heard that breast cancer risks are higher for women who have not given birth than for women who have, or that giving birth at a younger age reduces a woman's breast cancer risk. In this section, in addition to the epidemiologic guidelines listed at the beginning of this chapter, it's important to consider the effects of heterogeneity (mixed group). Earlier in this book I discussed how misleading study results can be when the effects of heterogeneity are ignored for women who have a family history of breast cancer (chapter 2) or are diagnosed with benign breast disease (chapter 5). Similarly, there are many different reasons why a woman may be childless or not have a child until she is older. For example, did a woman use birth control carefully until she was 33 and then conceive one month later? If so, how does this woman's risk compare to that of another who tried to become pregnant for years before finally conceiving at age 33? Or has a woman not given birth because her mate had a low or absent sperm count? How does this woman's risk compare to that of someone who failed to conceive either because her tubes were blocked or because she had a hormone imbalance that impeded a successful pregnancy? As you can see, if we consider risk to all of these women as a single group, we will not be able to identify subgroups that may have different risks due to different biological causes.

A recent study suggests that some types of infertility may be associated with an increase in breast cancer risk. In this study, women who said they had *no* fertility problem and who were older at the time of their first birth were not at increased risk of breast cancer compared to women who were less than 20 when their first child was born.[4] However, those who reported a "fertility problem" and whose first child was born after age 30 had a statistically significant increase in breast cancer risk compared to women whose first birth occurred before age 20.

Women with a fertility problem who first gave birth after 35 were three times more likely to be diagnosed with breast cancer as women whose first birth occurred before 20. The magnitude of the risk makes it more likely that the increased risk was due to their fertility problem. However, fewer than 50 women were present in each of the study groups. The small numbers and the lack of specificity about the types of infertility that might have been present make it difficult to apply these results meaningfully to all women with a fertility problem. This is clearly an area in which more research is needed.

As a group, women who gave birth to a first child at older ages, or even those who have not given birth, do not have statistically significant increases in breast cancer risk compared to women who gave birth at younger ages. Some studies find a small increase that might be due to factors not related to reproductive history. The possible effect of different types of infertility on breast cancer risk is currently unknown.

Childbirth and Family History of Breast Cancer

In several studies women who had a mother or sister with breast cancer and who first gave birth to a child at older ages did *not* have a statistically significant increase in breast cancer risk compared to women with a similar family history whose first child was born at younger ages. The number of women in these studies is small, and paternal history was not taken into account, so these results are not definitive. It is important to keep in mind that risks derived from groups with small numbers are far less secure than those derived from groups with larger numbers.

In one study of women who had two or more close relatives with breast cancer, those who first gave birth after age 24 did not have a higher risk than women with similar family histories who gave birth to a first child before age 24. Women who had a close relative with *bilateral* breast cancer and whose first child was born after age 24 did have a higher risk than those who were younger at the time of their first birth. The numbers in each of these groups were, however, too small to produce results that can be applied to all women with such a family history.[5]

Studies of women with BRCA and other mutations that increase hereditary cancer risk will be needed to determine whether childbearing history influences risk in this group. To date, studies do not find that the effects of a woman's risk due to family history and her risk due to older age at first birth can be added or multiplied together to produce her actual risk. In fact, in one study women with a BRCA mutation who had given birth were *more* likely to be diagnosed with breast cancer than were women who had not given birth.[6] Although some of the differences in this study were statistically significant, none was even twofold, so other factors may have contributed to the difference between the groups. The Gail model, a much-used tool for assessing breast cancer risk that is discussed in chapter 9, assumes that a woman's overall risk can be obtained by multiplying separate risks, such as family history and reproductive history.

Fertility Drugs

Women who have taken fertility drugs often have questions about how these drugs might have affected their breast cancer risk. The treatments are new, and the types, dose, and amount of time the drugs were used differ from person to person. These differences make any definitive assessment of fertility drug use and breast cancer risk impossible at the present time.[7] However, to date, there is no evidence that these drugs increase breast cancer risk to a consequential extent. In fact, most of the few available studies find no increase in risk.[8] Studies that do show an increase in risk include very few women, usually find an increase in risk to only premenopausal women, and have relative risks that are less than threefold.

Breast-Feeding

Few studies are available on breast-feeding, particularly long-term breast-feeding, for women in the United States. Most studies compare women who have ever breast-fed with those who have never breast-fed. Obviously, this comparison may not show the benefit of long-term breast-feeding, since the ever category includes women who breast-fed for only a short time. It is a heterogeneous group.

In several studies women who breast-fed four or more months had a slight but statistically significant decrease in risk of *premenopausal* breast cancer.[9] No difference was found for postmenopausal breast cancer risk, where larger numbers of women were included. In several other studies even women who breast-fed two or more years had no difference in breast cancer risk compared to women who did not breast-feed at all. However, very few women breast-fed for two or more years, so these results are not definitive.[10]

In one study, women who were "unsuccessful" in breast-feeding had a threefold increase in premenopausal breast cancer risk that was statistically significant.[11] The reasons for the failure to breast-feed were not given and the result is based on fewer than 50 women who developed breast cancer. This is an area in which we need larger studies that specify the reasons why a woman did not breast-feed.

As a group, these studies suggest that with modern, usually limited, breast-feeding practices, breast cancer risk is not appreciably decreased in women who breast-feed. The results of these studies in no way negate the many other benefits of breast-feeding to mother and child, however.

Age at Menopause

We hear a lot about "the years that a woman is exposed to estrogen" and the increase in breast cancer risk that is said to accompany an older age at menopause. However, in studies of women who start menopause at different ages, it's hard to find a difference in breast cancer risk that would be meaningful to an individual woman. For example, four studies compared women whose menopause occurred before age forty with women who were older at menopause. Those who were age fifty and older at the start of menopause were at significantly increased risk in only one of the four studies—and that risk was less than threefold. In the other three studies even women who started menopause at fifty-four and older had no statistically significant increase in risk.[12] Women who either entered menopause naturally or who had surgical menopause after age 45 also did not have a higher breast cancer risk than women whose menopause began at younger ages.[13]

Diet

Whole books have been written about the influence of diet on a woman's breast cancer risk. Everywhere you turn you hear stories about what to eat or what to avoid eating to reduce risk or even to prevent breast cancer. One day it's soy products, then fat, then phytoestrogens. Here I will briefly review some of what is and is not currently known scientifically about breast cancer risk and diet. As you will see, the evidence is still sketchy.

You might wonder why we don't know more about the effects of diet on breast cancer risk. However, if you think about what is involved in constructing such studies, you will quickly realize that diet is a very difficult topic to investigate. Few of us can remember what we ate last year, much less ten or fifteen years ago. A woman's diet over the years is likely to be more important than her eating habits of the last few months or even the last year, so lack of precise recall is a real impediment. However, even when people attempt to scrupulously report what they are eating, they are often not accurate reporters of what and how much they consume. Some believe that diet during the childhood and teen years may be crucial. All of these elements make it difficult to construct studies and interpret the effects of various aspects of a woman's diet on her risk of developing breast cancer.

In general, women (and men) who live in countries where the fat consumption is high have a greater breast cancer risk than individuals who live in countries where the fat consumption is lower. Since not all people in a country receive an equal share of the fat consumed in it, these studies are necessarily imprecise. There's another problem: the amount of fat a person consumes is probably an indicator of many other aspects of her lifestyle. These other aspects may have more (or as much) to do with a person's breast cancer risk than the fat in her diet.

Another complication in studying fat consumption arises because there are different kinds of fat. Some studies show, for example, that in countries where olive oil consumption is high, individuals have a lower risk of breast cancer than those who live in countries where the consumption of butter-fat is high. One study demonstrates just how complex this area can be.[14] It investigated the effect of both cooking method and the animal's diet on the amount of fat in beef. Grain-fed beef contained far more fat than grass-fed beef, no matter how it was cooked. Cooking greatly reduced the amount of fat in grain-fed beef but did little to reduce the amount in beef that was grass-fed. Even well-cooked beef that was grain-fed contained more fat than grass-fed beef, regardless of cooking style. So, in addition to cooking method, one needs to know how the animal was fed to be able to estimate the amount of fat in a serving of beef.

Then, there is the issue of the epidemiologic method itself, which, as you may remember, measures association, not cause and effect. Some years ago scientists were busily studying fat consumption and its possible effect on breast cancer risk. They soon realized that when people ate less fat, they tended to increase their consumption of foods that were high in fiber. One theory was that fiber might help to protect a woman from breast cancer. Different types of fiber were studied to see if some might be more protective than others. It appeared that some might be. Still later, the investigations focused on vitamins A, C, and E that are generally present in foods that are high in fiber. It seems that higher amounts of fiber intake may not directly influence breast cancer risk. Instead, fiber intake may be a marker for increased consumption of vitamins and other factors that do influence breast cancer risk.

Recent studies have investigated the effects of oxygen free radicals. These chemicals, which are formed as breakdown products of the foods we eat, are thought to damage the cells' DNA and in so doing increase cancer risk. The focus then became one of finding foods that were high in factors that could deactivate oxygen free radicals and so prevent damage to the cell. And so it goes—there are many interesting possibilities, but no firm results.

Here I'll mention just one more complication in studying diet: individual differences. Some people seem to require more of a dietary element than others to feel well and perhaps to reduce cancer risk. You may want to look back at figure 4 in chapter 3 at this point to see how individual differences might influence cancer risk. Until scientists have ways of measuring individual needs for dietary factors and individual differences in metabolizing foods, the results of even large studies may not have much to contribute to information about a particular individual's risk.

What's a reasonable person to do in the face of this changing and still uncertain information? My own approach is to use common sense and to hedge my bets by eating a balanced diet that is high in fresh fruits and vegetables and low in animal fat. In a way, eating such a balanced diet is defensive: no matter what future studies may show, you will have been eating some of the essential elements all along. At the same time, you have the satisfaction of feeling good and knowing that you are helping your body to function well and take care of you as only your body knows how. Let me quickly add here that this is a personal approach and is not based on definitive information about dietary elements that are effective in reducing cancer risk. I might also add that my bias is to eat with people I love and like.

Alcohol Consumption

Studies on alcohol consumption suffer from some of the same problems as studies on diet: they are based on individual reporting and not actual consumption patterns, with individual reporting notoriously unreliable. To interpret the results of studies on alcohol consumption and breast cancer risk, you need to know that the average bottle or can of beer contains about 13 grams of alcohol, a glass of wine about 11 grams, and a shot of liquor about 15 grams.[15] Obviously you can put more or less wine in a glass or buy differently sized bottles of beer; these are averages.

One study received a great deal of attention when it reported that women who consumed five or more grams of alcohol a day in beer, wine, or liquor had a significantly increased breast cancer risk.[16] This study assessed risk to women who consumed five or more grams of alcohol as one group. That is, women who drank less than half a bottle of beer or half a glass of wine a day were included with those who were very heavy drinkers and alcoholics. By including moderate and heavy drinkers in the same group, the study obscured information about moderate drinkers. This is another example of the type of misleading information that can be generated when heterogeneity is not taken into account. The increase in breast cancer risk was small—less than twofold, which suggests that other factors may well have been responsible for the difference that was present among the groups.

A more recent study investigated the effects of alcohol consumption by comparing breast cancer risk in non-drinkers and women who drank the following amounts each day: up to 5 grams, from 5 to 15 grams, and 15 or more grams of alcohol.[17] No significant difference in risk was present, even when heavier drinkers were compared to non-drinkers. Similar comparisons were made between non-drinkers and those who consumed up to 1, 1 to 3, or 3 or more drinks of beer, wine, or hard liquor a week. Again, women with different drinking habits did not differ in their breast cancer risk.

An analysis of six studies assessed breast cancer risk to women whose daily alcohol consumption was up to 1.5 grams, 1.5 grams to less than 5 grams, 5 grams to less than 15 grams, 15 grams to less than 30 grams, 30 grams to less than 60 grams, and 60 or more grams.[18] In *only four of the forty* comparisons did drinkers have a higher risk of breast cancer that was statistically significant. The heaviest drinkers were *not* those who had statistically different risks and none was even a twofold increase in risk—far less than the threefold or greater increase in the epidemiologic guidelines. As a group, these six study results do not show an increase in breast cancer risk to moderate (or even heavy drinkers) compared to non-drinkers.

In studies on alcohol consumption as a whole, risks of breast cancer to women who consume moderate amounts of alcohol are either not increased or are not increased to a measurable extent—which does not at all negate the sometimes profoundly harmful effects of immoderate alcohol consumption on many individuals' physical and psychosocial well-being.

Oral Contraceptives

& The risk of breast cancer to women who use oral contraceptives has been studied extensively. In most studies, no statistically significant increases in risk were found. In the relatively few instances in which a difference in risk is statistically significant, the relative risks are almost always less than three. And, as I will show you, the absolute risks are very small.

A 1996 study by a group called the Collaborative Group on Hormonal Factors in Breast Cancer reanalyzed data from 54 studies on oral contraceptive (OC) use. In the many factors considered—such as length of use, a woman's age when she first stared using OCs, and so forth—few of the differences between users and nonusers were statistically significant.[19] All of the relative risks were small (less than twofold), which means that other factors, not OCs, might be responsible for the differences in risk. This study contained such large numbers of women that some quite rightly argued that even small differences in risk were sufficient to show that OC use did, indeed, influence a woman's breast cancer risk in a substantial way. Let's take a closer look.

In this study, the breast cancers found in OC users were "less advanced clinically than the cancers diagnosed in never users" even twenty years after OC use stopped. The more favorable breast cancers in women who used OCs suggest that their breast cancers tended to be found at smaller sizes than those of the nonusers. (As I discussed in chapter 2, smaller breast cancers are generally less aggressive and are less likely to spread than larger breast cancers.) The difference in breast cancers between users and nonusers further suggests that these two groups have different lifestyles; that is, they differ from each other in more than just their OC use. These other differences, including prompter breast cancer detection, could also account for differences in breast cancer risk found between them.

To me, this is an elegant confirmation of the benefit of adhering to epidemiologic criteria in assessing results and being cautious about accepting as meaningful a result that does not adhere to these criteria—at least for evaluating an individual woman's risk. Sometimes small differences in population risks give scientists clues about fruitful areas for future investigations. Unfortunately, sometimes these small differences, which are important to scientists because they suggest future areas for investigation, are treated as if they have importance to an individual woman's risk.

But what if these small statistically significant differences in risk in this study *are* evidence that OCs increase breast cancer risk? In this large study, what was the absolute breast cancer risk to OC users? It turns out that the actual number of additional breast cancers that would be found in women who take OCs compared to women who never take them is so small that they were reported not as the number affected per hundred or even per thousand women, but the number likely to be affected as per 10,000 women. Even per 10,000 women, the additional numbers of breast cancers that might be found are small. Breast cancer risk increases with age, so the chances of finding breast cancers in older women who took OCs was higher than that of younger users. The additional number of breast cancers expected to be found *over fifteen years* ranged from 1.5 for women taking OCs from age 20 to 24 to 32 cases per 10,000 for women taking OCs from age 40 to 44. (In percentages these are risks of 0.015% to 0.32% spread over fifteen years.) Risks this small are unlikely to be of much or any concern to an individual.

Mortality

Women who use OCs are no more likely to die of breast cancer than women who do not use them.[20] In fact, in several studies, women who used birth control pills were half as likely to die of breast cancer compared to nonusers. Women using OCs may be more carefully followed by their doctors than other women. Therefore, early breast cancer detection, not pill use, may play a role in reducing breast cancer deaths. Whatever the reason, the finding is most important: *birth control pill use does not increase a woman's chances of dying of breast cancer,* and in some studies it is associated with a decreased risk of death.

Dose

Dose is a most important element in establishing cause. If OCs increase breast cancer risk, women who used pills with higher levels of hormones would be expected to have a higher breast cancer risk than women whose pills contained less. The hormone dose in OCs has decreased considerably since they were first widely used in the 1960s. The effect of hormone dose on breast cancer risk can be obtained by comparing breast cancer risk to women who first used the pill twenty or more years ago with more recent users. In the large Collaborative Group study, those who used OCs twenty or more years ago were not at higher risk than more recent users. Breast cancer risk therefore does not appear to be influenced by the amount of hormones in OCs.

Years of Use

A number of studies have investigated breast cancer risk to women who use OCs for ten and even fifteen years. In most studies women's risks don't increase with longer use, even when those who used older, higher dose pills are included.[21] In the large Collaborative Group study, the greatest increases in breast cancer occurred in women who used OCs for less than five or for five to nine years. In this time frame most or all of the breast cancers that were found were already present when the women started using OCs.

As you may remember, the women who took OCs had less advanced breast cancers than nonusers, so it is likely that the increase in risk is largely due to better early detection among OC users, not promotion of breast cancer by OCs. If OC use *had* promoted the growth of breast cancer, we would expect users to have more rapidly growing, more aggressive breast cancers than nonusers, instead of the more clinically favorable (slower growing, less aggressive) breast cancers that were found.

Family History of Breast Cancer

Several studies find that women who have a mother or sister with breast cancer are not at further increased risk if they take birth control pills, even when they use them for fifteen or more years.[22] In another study, OC users who had a mother or sister with breast cancer were not at increased risk of breast cancer if they used oral contraceptives for five or more years, but those with fewer years of use did have an increase in risk.[23] The cancers found in the first five years were present, of course, before OC use started. A recent study found no significant increase in risk to OC users who carried a BRCA mutation. However, 17 or fewer women were in each group studied, so these results are not definitive. Most studies on OC use and family history of breast cancer are based on small numbers of women and do not include paternal history, so more research is needed in this area as a whole.

Young Age at Diagnosis

In a number of studies, women who use birth control pills do not have an increased chance of developing breast cancer before age 40. These studies have very few women in them, since a breast cancer diagnosis at such a young age is quite rare. In the Collaborative Group study that used results from 54 studies, a slight increase in risk was found in young women in the first five years of use, but not later. These women's breast cancers were likely to have been present before OC use began, since breast cancers generally grow eight to twelve years before they are detected. Surveillance was probably more thorough in the users than nonusers, leading to a higher detection rate in OC users.

One study found that compared to nonusers, OC users had a threefold increase in breast cancer risk from age 30 to 34. Because the relative risk was over three and was statistically significant, the increase in risk is unlikely to be due to other differences between users and nonusers, and appeared to be due to OC use. Before you become too concerned, let's take a look at what this statistically significant increase in risk is in absolute terms. It turns out that the 3.3-fold increase is an absolute risk of *one in 7,000 a year*.[24] Because so few women develop breast cancer before age 34, a threefold increase in risk was a very small actual risk.

Age at First Use

Does a woman's age when she first started using the pill influence her breast cancer risk? Most studies find no increase in risk to those who started using OCs when they were young. In the large Collaborative Group study, no increases in risk were found after five years of use, even for women who started using birth control pills before age 20.

Among women whose OC use began at very young ages there is a subgroup that did so to help with hormone imbalance. This subgroup *might* have an increase in breast cancer risk. If so, their inclusion in the overall group who started OC use at 16 or younger would produce a slight risk to the group as a whole—another example of heterogeneity. This is a group that deserves further study, with emphasis on a woman's reason for starting OC use.

Use before First Pregnancy

A number of studies have investigated the risk of breast cancer to young women who started using OCs before their first pregnancy. Studies of women who developed breast cancer before age 45 have had small numbers, but most find no increase in risk, even with eight years of use.[25]

Summary of Oral Contraceptive Use and Breast Cancer Risk

As a group, the many studies on oral contraceptive use and breast cancer risk are reassuring. Women who use OCs are not more likely to die of breast cancer. OC users who do develop breast cancer, even twenty years after OC use stops, have *less clinically advanced* cancers than women who never use them. No increase in breast cancer risk to women who use OCs for even fifteen years is seen in most studies. In one large study where absolute numbers of breast cancers were estimated based on small but statistically significant increases in relative risks, the extra numbers of breast cancers found in OC users were so small they were reported in terms of 10,000 women and over a period of fifteen years.

Key Points to Remember

- Women who differ in various aspects of their reproductive history (age at menarche, age when their first child was born, not giving birth at all, use of fertility drugs, breast-feeding, and age at menopause) either have no statistically significant increase in breast cancer risk or have such small increases that they may well be due to other causes, not reproductive history.
- Diet is difficult to study in a way that can be applied to an individual, so to date there is no definitive evidence about specific dietary factors that increase or reduce breast cancer risk.
- Moderate alcohol consumption does not appear to increase a woman's breast cancer risk.
- Women who use oral contraceptives are not at significantly increased risk of developing breast cancer in most studies, even with fifteen or more years of use.
- Women who use oral contraceptives do not have an increased chance of dying of breast cancer.
- In one large study the absolute increases in breast cancer risk to OC users were so small they were reported per 10,000 women over a fifteen-year period. Risks this small are unlikely to be relevant to an individual woman's decision making about OC use.

Concluding Comments about Part II

Now that you have read the risk information in Part II, you may well be asking yourself why it sometimes differs from other accounts you have heard and read. How can you determine which information about a risk is correct? Actually, it's not that other accounts are necessarily "wrong." Instead, much of any difference may be due to the format or perspective. Just as a mountain's appearance changes, depending on whether you are twenty miles away or at its base, risk information can also seem quite different depending on the format in which it is presented.

The risk information that you read about in Part II was presented in terms that are likely to be relevant to an individual who is interested in making reasonable health care decisions. You may remember that for risk information to be useful, it should include:

- A time frame in which the risk occurred. For example, as you saw in chapter 2, the average woman's breast cancer risk is 1 in 9, or 11% from age 20 to 80, but is 2% from age 20 to 50. As a woman goes through each year without a diagnosis of breast cancer, she leaves that risk behind.
- The use of actual (absolute) risk instead of a comparison of one group's risk to that of another's. For example, as you saw in chapter 5, the same breast cancer risk to women with atypical ductal hyperplasia can be presented either as a relative risk of 3 or as a risk of less than 1 percent a year.
- Consideration of the possible effects of heterogeneity. For example, as explained in chapter 2, women with similar-appearing family histories can have very different breast cancer risks, since some have an in-

creased hereditary risk and others do not. In studying a mixed group as a single entity, differences in risks to subgroups may be obscured.

In Part II you also learned about criteria that epidemiologists have developed to assess the likelihood that an agent (such as a potential risk factor) causes a disease and is not merely present in the study group for extraneous reasons. As discussed in chapter 6, an agent is more likely to be causal when:

- Exposure to it occurs before the onset of the disease,
- It is associated with similar risks in a number of studies,
- An effect of dose on disease rate can be shown,
- Statistically significant differences in risk are present, and
- The group exposed to the agent has at least a three- to fourfold increase or decrease in risk, compared to the nonexposed group.

Although these formats and criteria are not complex and rely largely on common sense, they do take time to explain in a meaningful fashion and require some focus in attention before they can be understood. We are living in an era in which the mass media and even medical and scientific journals present information as increasingly smaller sound and visual "bites." Our society generates an amazing pressure to get to the point of a story quickly, to "encapsulate" it, to reduce it to a pill which may, without much thought or investigation, be "swallowed whole."

This push to "get to the point" may lead the media and physicians— two main sources of risk information—to provide shorter, sparer descriptions and to use generalizations, which in turn can lead to confusion and misunderstanding. For example, as you saw in chapter 6, even if one accepts the 30% to 50% increase in breast cancer risk that is reported in some studies on hormone replacement therapy, this is an absolute increase of only 0.6 cases of breast cancer per 100 women from age 50 to 70. By presenting the same study result in a different format or without using epidemiologic criteria to assess it, the same finding may generate very different levels of concern.

Physicians are not exempt from pressures to get to the point in discussing risk. Their time with each patient is diminishing (an average of 13.6 to 16.5 minutes in one recent study[1]) and they are not usually trained in or comfortable with epidemiology and statistics. According to an article in the highly respected British medical journal *The Lancet,* the training physicians receive may also engender a sense of unease when they lack information or are uncertain: "Traditional medical education has fostered . . . the notion that uncertainty is a manifestation of ignorance, weakness, or failure."[2] To save time and to avoid feeling uncertain, physicians may simplify an issue or a risk. In time, the simplification, the generalization—such as a reliance on relative risk instead of absolute risk—can be mistaken by both doctor and patient for the complete picture.

Many of us, not just physicians, may, without realizing it, slip into thinking about risk in a generalized, overly simplistic fashion that is less useful in individual decision making than a more comprehensive approach would be. As you read Part III, I suggest that you keep in mind the quotation cited above and remember also that physicians are trained in medicine, not in cancer risk assessment or in making prophecies about the future. The points I've just discussed may help to explain why information about breast cancer risk factors is often simplified and generalized, and may also help you to better interpret what you hear from physicians as you apply what you have learned in Part II in setting up your own breast health program—the subject of Part III.

Part III

USING THE FACTS

EIGHT

Navigating the Medical System

Now that you have read about various breast cancer risks and have learned what to look for to determine whether or not a risk is likely to be large enough to be important to you, the next step is to obtain the breast health care you want. In this chapter I'll discuss ways to help you effectively use the medical system to achieve that goal, including:

- Types of breast health specialists you might consult
- Elements of effective doctor-patient interactions
- Second opinions
- Ways to find a compatible doctor
- Reactions of some physicians to risk information

Specialists and Their Roles

The extraordinary growth of medical information and the development of new technologies have made it increasingly difficult for any one health professional to be completely informed about all aspects of breast care. This in turn has led to increasing specialization. No longer is it reasonable to expect any one physician to be able to direct all of your breast care. By working with a number of different specialists, such as a nurse, nurse practitioner, radiologist, gynecologist, surgeon, and pathologist, each responsible for a specific area, you are more likely to have access to the latest advances. However, unless you have an understanding of the contribution each can make, the medical approach to your breast care might seem fragmented and confusing.

The following is a brief description of the responsibilities of the health professionals who can help you with a breast concern or a breast problem. The specialist is listed in the order that you might encounter him or her if you were to have a breast lump, pain, thickening, or discharge.

- *Gynecologist, internist, family practice doctor, nurse, nurse practitioner*

A nurse or a physician in one of these specialties is often the first to learn about or to detect a woman's breast lump or other breast symptom. In such cases a woman is usually referred to a radiologist for a mammogram and to a surgeon for further examination.

- *Mammography technologist*

These health professionals are responsible for the appropriate placement of a woman's breasts when a mammogram is taken so that as much of the breast as possible is included in the film and a clear image is obtained. This often overlooked group plays an important role and is increasingly trained to answer questions about mammography and other related issues.

- *Radiologist*

These doctors read and interpret mammograms, and so may detect calcifications or a distortion in breast architecture that warrants further investigation, even when no change can be felt in a physical examination. Radiologists also perform "localization" procedures in which a precise area of the breast is bracketed or marked so that small amounts of tissue can be removed, either by the radiologist or the surgeon.

- *Surgeon*

Surgeons are perhaps best known for performing surgery, but this is not the only service they provide. Women who feel at high risk of breast cancer may derive great comfort by having a surgeon examine their breasts regularly. Then, if they should develop a breast problem they will not be looking for a new doctor during a time of stress.

- *Pathologist*

Pathologists examine breast tissue or breast fluid under a microscope to determine the types of cells that are present and their extent. Increasingly, pathologists also perform laboratory tests on breast cells to look for the presence of alterations such as Her-2 neu, a marker for an aggressive type of breast cancer (described in chapter 3). These markers, in conjunction with information about the type of cancer cell and the size of the tumor, can provide additional information about the most useful treatments and about prognosis. *Modern-day treatment decisions by the other breast specialists are made on the basis of the pathologist's findings.* For this reason, as I'll discuss later, a second opinion by a pathologist can be particularly useful.

- *Radiation oncologist*

If breast cancer is found, women see a radiation oncologist to discuss whether radiation treatment might be helpful in their situation. Radiation therapy is used to control cancer in the breast, the chest area, and surrounding tissue.

- *Medical oncologist*

Following a breast cancer diagnosis, women see a medical oncologist to discuss whether chemotherapy or other agents, such as tamoxifen, would be of help in controlling cancer cells that might have traveled from the breast to other parts of the body.

- *Plastic surgeon*

These specialists can provide breast reconstruction to women who have a mastectomy. Women often visit several and ask to see photographs of previous breast reconstructions that the doctor has completed.

It is important to be clear about the role of these different specialists, and to remember that no one doctor is responsible for providing all of the help in diagnosing or treating a breast problem or breast cancer.

Effective Interactions with Doctors

❧ Many people tell me they want the doctor to think they are handling their medical concern well and that they are not "complainers." These individuals strive to be cheerful in the doctor's presence, even when their spirits are low. They may be reluctant to tell their doctor when they don't understand, when they have questions, when they forget information, when they would like more of the doctor's time, or even when they are uncomfortable with a suggestion their doctor has made. This reticence is unfortunate. Often I find that when I encourage a woman to let her doctor know what is troubling her or what she would like, she discovers with pleasure that the doctor wants to help and is ready to provide more information. Obviously doctors can be more effective when they are aware of the specifics of their patients' questions and concerns.

Sometimes misunderstandings arise between a woman and her physician because she isn't aware of some of the elements that shape the physician's approach. The following sections contain examples that have helped my patients to understand and to interact with their physicians in a more meaningful fashion. As you read them, you might want to keep pen and paper handy in order to write down other ways that might be useful to you in your own situation.

Keeping Up, Keeping Calm

Medical care, technology, and the information base itself are all in a state of rapid change. Physicians increasingly feel overworked, are finding their incomes diminished, and express concerns about losing control of the type of care they want their patients to have. Most spend less time with each patient and have less time to learn about new developments than they would like. Even though information is growing at a tremendous rate, few mechanisms are in place to help doctors sort through it or integrate it into their clinical practices.

Physicians often tell me that they don't have time to process new information to see how it fits into their clinical practice and lack the time and expertise to track down and evaluate details of the many studies that are published. Insufficient time affects all areas of doctor-patient interaction, so keep that in mind as you read the following sections.

Scheduling

Let's take a look at the scheduling of appointments from the physician's point of view. Not only do doctors have less time for their patients these days (about 15 minutes per visit), but patients are now more likely to expect doctors to be aware of and to discuss information they have gleaned from articles, books, and the Internet. From the doctor's medical perspective, some of the patient's questions and even the information she has found in an article or on the Internet may be irrelevant to that person's treatment or follow-up plan, and may make the doctor's already overly crowded day even busier, without helping the patient. Both doctor and patient may wind up with a sense of being rushed and yet may still not be able to satisfactorily cover the (different) areas of importance to each.

In a study of over one thousand patient visits with physicians, only 9% of all discussions physicians held with patients provided sufficient information to enable patients to make informed decisions.[1] When decisions involved intermediate or complex areas, fewer than 1% of the discussions were complete. The investigators in this study, most of whom were physicians, concluded:

> By the most minimal definition consistent with an ethical framework, decision making in clinical practice may fall short of a basic level of patient involvement in routine decisions.[2]

Time constraints may account for some of this lack of discussion and failure to involve the patient in a meaningful way.

To enable the doctor's office to schedule time that is sufficient for you to receive the information and help that you want:

- Be sure to ask for a longer appointment when you know you have areas you want to discuss in depth. If your doctor's office is unwilling to schedule more time with you, you may want to think about finding another who will. Also, be sure to ask about the fee for a longer visit so that you are not surprised by it.
- Write down your main questions or concerns and take them with you—leave plenty of space around the items on the list so you can easily write in the answers while you are there or shortly after you leave. During the visit, have the list in front of you so you can look at it during the visit to help keep the discussion focused on the issues of most concern to you.
- Consider sending some of your major questions to the doctor in advance so he or she will have time to think about them and do any necessary research before your visit.
- Try grouping your questions around your major areas of concern so that you can begin to sort out areas of greater and lesser importance.
- Remember to ask the doctor which questions or issues are most

important from his or her perspective, and why this is so. The "why" part is sometimes as or more informative than the response. Ask yourself if the "why" part makes sense to you and is congruent with your values or aims.

- If, after thinking about the doctor's answers to your questions *and the reasons for them,* you still are not clear about the information, be sure to schedule another visit and prepare a second series of questions. Complex issues may take several rounds of visits for you to achieve clarity.

Remember, the doctor is your employee. He or she is there to provide the help and information you want. Your role is to be as clear as you can be about what you need and want, and to be ready to learn, think, and ponder so you can be even more clear at the next visit. The doctor's role is to help meet your needs and objectives by providing information and services.

Framing

In this time of increased specialization and shortened visits, the way you frame your concerns and ask questions of doctors may determine the answers you get, even from the very best and most dedicated physicians. For example, many women recently diagnosed with atypical hyperplasia, DCIS, or LCIS quite naturally ask their doctor if surgical removal of the area will prevent them from developing cancer in the future (see chapter 5 for a discussion of these breast cell types). They may then be shaken to hear the doctor say that they certainly could develop breast cancer in the future. On the basis of such statements, some women conclude that they would be wise to have a mastectomy.

When I inquire, I learn that these women have asked if cancer *could* occur. When the question is asked in this way, there is only one honest response: "Yes, it could." But what my patients actually meant to ask their doctor was something like, "Is a biopsy or lumpectomy generally useful in situations like mine? How likely is it that cancer will occur in the future if I choose that option?" "How reliable are the studies in this area?" Once these women stop and reflect, they realize that even without their recently diagnosed breast condition a breast cancer could occur, and even after prophylactic mastectomy, as described in chapter 10. The point is to be sure you ask a question in such a way that you will receive specific information, not generalizations that may appear to be grim forebodings.

Worried Doctor Syndrome

The term *breast cancer prevention* is often loosely used—so often, in fact, that both patients and doctors may begin to feel or to act as if a doctor's role is to keep a woman from ever getting breast cancer. Since no one knows how to prevent cancer, this can lead to what I call the "Worried Doctor Syndrome." For example, a number of physician colleagues have expressed concern about prescribing tamoxifen to women without a breast cancer diagnosis as a way of "preventing" breast cancer or reducing breast cancer risk. These physicians tell me they are unsure that their patients will receive any appreciable benefit from tamoxifen (for some of the reasons discussed in chapter 10) and express concern about the well-documented increase in risk of uterine cancer, cataracts, blood clots, and other problems women who take tamoxifen may have.

These doctors are also concerned about the emotional and legal consequences if they advise a woman not to take tamoxifen and she later develops breast cancer. Will she blame her doctor? Remember, those who become doctors tend to do so because they want to help people. They do not want their patients to be angry with them or even upset with them. One physician told me:

> Sometimes I feel caught. It seems that what a patient is asking is if something might possibly help. I can see that based on what we know now it probably won't help or will help her very little. And it may even cause her harm. But if I tell her not to do it and then she gets cancer, she could blame me.

Another said:

> If I see a woman who is at high risk of breast cancer I better do *something*. I feel I either need to tell her to have her breasts taken off or take tamoxifen. If I tell her not to do anything, or maybe if I don't suggest something, I could be in trouble later. Tamoxifen may be easier for her to tolerate than mastectomy. And I know too that with tamoxifen I might be making her miserable for nothing.

It is this urge to do *something* that needs to be scrutinized, especially given the excellent prognosis a woman has when her breast cancer is found at a small size. So remember, when a drug or procedure is mentioned, suggested, or even recommended, ask yourself questions such as the following: Is this for me? What do *I* want? Will this procedure (drug or other approach) help reduce *my* anxiety, or my relatives', or my doctor's? In absolute risk terms, how great a difference will this suggested approach make this year, in five years, and in ten years? If your risk will be reduced by only a small amount in five years, you may want to wait several years to see what studies show at that time, particularly if the suggested approach is new.

Indirect Advice

Doctors, particularly when they are unsure or have no strong opinion about a drug or a treatment option, may not tell a patient directly what they think. Instead, they may offer several approaches as options, trying to be neutral and watching to see which the patient appears to prefer. Patients react in various ways to this approach. They may

- expect the doctor to make a decision for them and become angry or frightened when they are given options.
- believe the doctor wants them to choose the most "drastic" approach or it would never have been mentioned.
- believe the doctor is uninformed because he or she is not fully supporting information that was recently reported in the mass media.
- realize that not enough is known about the risks and benefits of the various approaches for the doctor to be able to recommend only one.

Instead of guessing, I encourage you to ask how your doctor perceives the pros and cons of each approach, given your particular situation.

"If I were your relative . . ."

To determine a doctor's best advice, some women ask doctors what they would suggest if she were a relative. This is not as useful an approach as you might initially think, since what may be appropriate for the doctor's relative may not be for you. Also, the relative may not take the doctor's advice! Betty, a 36-year-old patient of mine who had lumpy breasts, was not served at all by following the advice a doctor said he would give to his relative. She was at an anxious and uncertain time in her life, having just gone through an acrimonious divorce and some unsettling changes at work. Betty also worried that she would die of breast cancer, "just like my mother did before she was forty."

When Betty's doctors told her that her breasts were quite lumpy and that she had "fibrocystic disease" she became even more anxious. One doctor, largely in response to Betty's expressed anxiety, mentioned that prophylactic mastectomy was an option. She assumed that the doctor wouldn't bring up "such a drastic procedure" unless he thought she "really needed it," and then became even more concerned about her breast cancer risk. When she sought an opinion from another doctor he gave it promptly: "If you were my wife, I would advise you to have your breasts removed immediately." Betty told me later she thought his comments meant that she probably had breast cancer already. She scheduled surgery promptly.

I'll never forget the anguished phone call I received from Betty after both her breasts had been removed and she learned that no cancer was present in any of the breast tissue. She was not pleased (as some women are) that her breasts had been removed before cancer was present, since she had been firmly convinced that cancer was present before her surgery. Betty was unhappy with the way the implants felt, saying, "It doesn't feel like my body anymore." Her anxieties about breast cancer remained after the surgery and she continued to feel fragile. Betty became quite angry with the doctor who urged her to have the surgery, saying that he had "railroaded" her into it.

Betty's experience is a sad example of what can happen when a person is not clear about surgical outcomes and when she relies on others to make an important decision for her. Situations like hers are unfortunately not uncommon when a woman feels vulnerable due to the death of a loved one or to another unsettling life change. At these times women may make decisions that they later regret. In some cases actions that are not fully thought out result from "imprinting" (discussed below).

Imprinting

What I call imprinting can occur during an interaction between patient and physician at a time of high anxiety or intensity, as is often present when a woman has a breast lump or when atypical hyperplasia, an in situ cancer, or an invasive cancer is found. At these times, a person's emotional system may be particularly sensitive, so the words and even the demeanor of an authority figure such as a doctor can make a markedly strong imprint that lasts for months, even if her situation is later found to be quite different from the original doctor's pronouncement.

Virginia's experiences illustrate the effects of imprinting. She was 47 when atypical hyperplasia was found in her left breast. According to Virginia, the doctor told her that her risk of breast cancer was "greatly increased," that this was a "serious" condition, and that she "would be wise to schedule a mastectomy now." Fortunately Virginia saw another doctor who told her there was a 99% chance that she would not be diagnosed with breast cancer in the next year and that her breasts were fairly easy to follow by mammography and physical examination. The second doctor told Virginia that she could certainly have a mastectomy if she wished, but this was not her first recommendation.

When I initially met with Virginia she was in agony. She said:

> I keep waking up and hearing that doctor's [the first doctor's] words. I hear what you are saying and I hear what my new doctor is saying. It's as if there are two of me. One part of me is so scared and the other sees that my chances are pretty good. I can see intellectually it's not so bad. But it *feels* terribly frightening.

Virginia was suffering from an imprinting that occurred in her meeting with the first doctor. She heard and was imprinted by initially hearing that her condition was serious. When she later learned that her risks were not as great as she had first believed, and that she was not "doomed to get cancer," her intellect grasped the situation before her emotional system could follow. With time her emotional reactions and intellectual processes became more congruent, and she was able to feel comfortable with the follow-up program suggested by the second doctor. As you can imagine, problems sometimes arise when a woman acts while in the grip of imprinting. Not infrequently, six months or so may be needed to recover from it.

Spiral of Concern

In response to a sympathetic doctor with whom she feels comfortable, a woman may express her deepest, most frightening concerns about being diagnosed with breast cancer. In response to the *woman's* expressed fears, her doctor may discuss prophylactic mastectomy. The patient may (mistakenly) hear that prophylactic mastectomy is the doctor's primary recommendation and assume that her risk must be very high indeed, as was illustrated previously. She may then become even more concerned about her risk. When she expresses this now increased anxiety, the doctor's concern about her may also increase.

If this upward spiral of concern continues, the doctor may at some point conclude that this patient is so anxious that she *would* be better off having a prophylactic mastectomy. In such cases, a woman may have a prophylactic mastectomy (or other treatment) as a result of a spiral of concern that grew in intensity.

Second opinions and direct questions to the doctor about why he or she is making a recommendation can help to detect a growing spiral of concern. Specifically, ask the doctor whether the suggestion is:

- A recommendation based on studies. If so, how reliable is the scientific evidence? On what is it based?
- A recommendation based on the doctor's clinical experience. If so, what is it? On how many people is the recommendation based?
- One of several options. Is one approach clearly better than another?

The "Watchful Patient Syndrome"

My patients watch their doctors minutely and sometimes use subtle cues to decide, for example, that their doctor no longer likes them or thinks the situation is graver than it actually is. Marianne, a 43-year-old woman whose breasts were quite lumpy, called me in a panic one day to tell me she thought that her doctor had felt a cancer in her breast but didn't want to tell her until he was sure. She explained that when she went for a visit the doctor was very "serious" as he examined her breasts and didn't engage in his usual conversation with her. At the end of the exam he didn't smile or engage in talk, as was their usual custom. Instead, he reminded her that she was due for a mammogram and asked her to have it before her next appointment with him. "I think he couldn't bring himself to tell me," she said. "He looked so sad. He'll probably tell me about it after he sees the mammogram."

I knew Marianne's doctor, so I knew something she didn't: her doctor's wife was quite ill, and he was concerned about her. Test results on his wife were due back that day, so he was probably particularly tense. I discovered Marianne's doctor had not found anything worrisome in her exam. His demeanor had nothing to do with her. Misunderstandings of this type arise when a woman does not check up on the evidence. Marianne could have spared herself a great deal of worry by asking the doctor directly, "Did you find anything new or unusual in my breast exam?"

Second Opinions

These days many women seek second opinions—or third, or fourth—often from different specialists. This approach is useful, and even essential in some cases, but the process can also add to a person's sense of confusion. Here are some guidelines that may help to make your second opinion experience more comfortable and rewarding:

- See different types of specialists. The training and life experiences of medical specialists in different fields—for example, surgeons and radiation oncologists—often vary, leading to different perspectives and opinions. Access to alternative ways of thinking and approaches may round out your own thinking so that you can make a more informed decision.
- Ask why the physician thinks the way he or she does, and what evidence or study supports this view.
- Listen to your intuition or gut feeling. If what you are hearing doesn't seem right, feel right, or hang together in a way that makes sense to you, you may need more visits with that doctor and/or consultations with another doctor.
- Obtain your second opinion from a doctor who is in a different town or who is affiliated with a different hospital than the first. This will make it easier for the second doctor to disagree with the first without damaging his or her sources of future patients or risking hurt feelings from a colleague with whom the consulting doctor frequently interacts.
- If you have breast surgery, be sure to obtain a second pathology review from a pathologist who specializes in breast disease. The pathology report is like an architect's blueprint of a structure. It tells you

whether a castle or a cottage is present. Since other specialists' treatment recommendations are based on the pathologist's determination, *this may well be the most important second opinion you receive.*

I often see women who have consulted three different surgeons, a radiologist, a medical oncologist, and a radiation oncologist about a breast lump or breast cancer. These women have taken great care to choose physicians in each field who have known expertise with breast cancer. Yet very few have obtained a second pathology opinion from a pathologist who is specially trained in breast disease.

Jane's experience shows how important a second pathology opinion can be. When I first saw Jane, her husband, and her mother, they were distraught. Jane's breast lump had just been diagnosed as a very large invasive breast cancer. No cancer had been found in the lymph nodes under her arm, which was encouraging. Still, because of the size of the breast cancer, several doctors strongly suggested that she take chemotherapy. Jane was in her early thirties and did not yet have children, but hoped to have them. She feared that if she took chemotherapy it would put her into menopause and she would not be able to become pregnant. Her husband grimly said he had other concerns as well. To him her prognosis seemed quite bleak, even with chemotherapy.

At the time of the first visit I suggested that Jane consider obtaining a second pathology review. This review (and the third review she later obtained) differed substantially from the initial report. The later two pathologists found that most of Jane's large breast lump did *not* contain invasive cancer. Most of the tumor was composed of ductal carcinoma in situ. Only microscopic amounts of invasive disease were present. With this different finding, Jane's doctors no longer recommended chemotherapy. She and her family were elated to learn that instead of a 50% to 60% chance that her cancer would recur, it was now highly unlikely that it had spread. Jane has since had several children and has remained cancer free.

Finding a Doctor or Nurse

Now that you know about the types of medical specialists who help women with breast concerns and have considered ways that might help you to interact with doctors in a more effective manner, you may wonder how to go about finding the doctor or doctors for your breast health care. (Here I'll use the term "doctor" for doctor, nurse, or nurse practitioner, since nurses and nurse practitioners are involved in providing breast health care in many communities.) One of the best ways, of course, is to ask friends, relatives, and associates about their experiences with physicians and nurses. Remember that not all people work well together, so a doctor who suited one of your friends may not be appropriate for you. To find out, you'll need one or several visits.

If you have had frightening or discouraging visits with doctors in the past, you may want to avoid snap judgments about the new doctors you meet. Remember, your past experiences may be influencing you. However, if you continue to feel uncomfortable after several visits, you may want to look for another doctor.

Women often tell me that they "can't" see a particular doctor because he or she isn't on their medical plan. Of course they can see any doctor they choose—if they are willing to pay! For office visits the fee may be less than you thought, and you are certainly entitled to call ahead to learn what the fee would be. So, for peace of mind you may decide to pay to see a particular doctor or nurse several times a year, even if that health professional is not covered by your medical plan.

Remember, in choosing a doctor or nurse you are choosing someone to help you. The doctor is your employee and is being hired to provide a service that measures up to your expectations. If it does not, it is the doctor's responsibility to explain why he or she is not doing so. A truly healing doctor's role is to help you feel more in control, more comfortable, not less so. For this to happen, you have your role to play as well. Your responsibility is to communicate your situation as clearly as you can, to understand what your options are, to choose what seems best for you, and then be clear with yourself and with the doctor about what is helping you and what is not. You may also find it useful to maintain a sense of responsibility for yourself and not give up all your control or decision-making power.

In a healthy interaction each person accepts responsibility for her role, speaks up and asks questions when something is not clear, and presents information to others to give them a better understanding of her thoughts and actions. This approach can also work well with your doctor. Since the doctor cannot read your mind, he or she will be able to respond most usefully by receiving complete and accurate feedback from you.

Your Doctor and Risk Information

Medical information, particularly risk information, can be quite dense. The doctor can give information, hear the patient repeat it clearly, and assume that the patient understands it fully. At a later time a patient may ask why she wasn't told about an issue, only to learn that the doctor considered it a part of what was discussed. In my experience, people are most likely to understand the ramifications of information if they also receive background information, learn something of the conceptual framework so they have a better idea of where their questions do or don't fit into current medical thinking, have an opportunity to ask questions, and take time to talk to others about the issues. In this way they and those close to them can become aware of parts of the information that are not clear or that do not seem to be congruent. In some institutions nurses help people think through the implications of the information. Increasingly geneticists and genetic counselors are providing this help with regard to risk information, as I discuss in chapter 9.

In seeking risk information or advice about how to use risk information, remember also that physicians are trained to diagnose and treat illness. Your risk is not an illness! The doctor's training has not prepared him or her to see into the future with any greater certainty than you can yourself. Studies find that, as a group, physicians tend not to use risk information, even when it is available for a particular topic.[3] Physicians treat individuals, so it is not surprising that they are sometimes suspicious of results based on groups of people. Although decisions based on "actuarial or statistical" information generally provide more reliable results, physicians tend to be more comfortable with anecdotal evidence based on their own practices and experience than on the result of scientific studies.[4]

Each of these approaches—the anecdotal and the scientific—has its strengths and weaknesses. For example, anecdotal evidence is limited since it is based on relatively few people. Recent experiences or more difficult cases may be remembered more vividly than others. The scientific approach is usually based on a larger group, attempts to establish cause and effect, and is less likely to be swayed by exceptions than is anecdotal evidence. However, studies of groups may not take important individual differences into account or may obscure them, as when heterogeneity is present. And the results of a scientific study may be misinterpreted or misleading. Increasingly, the latest scientific evidence is being used to make decisions in clinical practice.

The lack of comfort with risk and statistics, coupled with the Worried Doctor Syndrome I discussed earlier in this chapter, can lead to a conflict of interest between patients and physicians that is not noticeable to either group. In an effort to provide as much help as possible, physicians may offer treatments involving all that their area of expertise can provide. For example, a surgeon may feel more comfortable if a woman has her breasts removed to prevent the occurrence of a future cancer. The physician knows full well that cancer can still occur after prophylactic mastectomy. If it should occur, however, it will be a rare occurrence. The surgeon will have done all that he or she can do and so won't feel remiss—as might be the case if no surgery were suggested and cancer were to occur. Or the medical oncologist or surgeon may suggest tamoxifen to reduce a woman's risk of future breast cancer, not fully appreciating how little the absolute reduction in risk actually is.

I don't mean to single out surgeons or medical oncologists here with these simple examples. Such an approach is only human. In my experience, most specialists (including geneticists) can have the same tendency, which originates in a sincere desire to help. This is why *your* evaluation of risk and the decisions you make in setting up a reasonable, responsible breast health program are so important. The follow-up or the treatment, after all, is for you and not for your doctor. The aim here is your comfort level, not your doctor's.

To help you make useful decisions about your breast care and followup, I present information about cancer risk assessment and genetic testing in chapter 9 and specific guidelines for making health care decisions about breast and ovarian cancer in chapter 10.

Key Points to Remember

☙ To be able to more effectively use the medical care system, remember:

- Several different medical specialists are generally needed to provide adequate breast health care.

- Call ahead to schedule extra time with your doctor if you will need a longer than usual appointment.
- Take written questions with you to your medical appointments, but also be prepared to talk about areas not covered by your questions, should you learn your questions are not relevant or not sufficiently comprehensive.
- Frame your questions in an organized and succinct manner to reflect your major areas of concern.
- The answers you receive may be determined by how you frame your questions.
- Doctors' recommendations are sometimes designed to reduce their own anxiety or to assure themselves that they are offering all that their specialty can provide.
- The emotional effects of information you received at a time of stress may persist in strong fashion, even when the initial information changes.
- Second opinions are useful, especially from a pathologist, if breast tissue is removed.
- Physicians are generally not trained to discuss risk, and in some cases tend to rely more on anecdotal evidence than on scientific studies.
- The doctor is your employee and is there to provide you with the care you want.

NINE

Cancer Risk Assessment
and Genetic Testing:
Are They for You?

For counselors the central issue in counseling is to provide the individual with an estimation of risk, while for the counselee it is what to do about a risk they already perceive to be high.[1]

As I hope I have made clear in this book so far, I strongly support a Cancer Risk Assessment process that includes helping individuals make a health plan that will help them to feel and to be as safe as possible. Risk information, by itself, is of little value to the individual unless it is applied in her health care. In this chapter I will discuss the workings of the Cancer Risk Assessment process—a process that includes helping women make use of the information they receive.

Who Benefits Most from Cancer Risk Assessment?

☙ I often receive calls from women asking if they would benefit by having a Cancer Risk Assessment. As you might expect, those who have a family history of cancer are most likely to be concerned about cancer risk. Some have concerns about their own health, some are curious about their risk, and some are worried about their children's risk.

Some people tell me they have waited years to make an appointment to investigate their cancer risk, since they fear what they might learn. I hope you now realize that Cancer Risk Assessment is actually a win-win process. Information you receive can help you to put aside concerns about a risk if you learn that it is not appreciably increased or is not as high as you had expected. Or, if you learn that your cancer risk is increased, you can make plans to protect yourself. Either way, you benefit.

I am frequently asked who "should" seek Cancer Risk Assessment. The answer is: anyone who has unresolved questions about risks, causes, and follow-up options. From my perspective the Cancer Risk Assessment process is not just for individuals who have a strong family history of cancer. It can also be quite useful if you have questions about your breast and other cancer risks that relate to:

- A personal history of cancer
- A diagnosis of benign breast disease, ductal carcinoma in situ, or lobular carcinoma in situ
- Use of hormone replacement therapy at menopause
- Birth control pill use
- Reproductive history factors, such as not having given birth to a child
- Diet and alcohol consumption
- Various environmental agents

Having questions about the origin of cancer is yet another good reason to seek Cancer Risk Assessment.

There are generalizations but no certainties in identifying who is most likely to have an increased risk of cancer due to strong hereditary factors. As you may remember from previous chapters, an increased hereditary risk is more likely in families where an individual is diagnosed at a young age, where several generations are affected, and where several different types of cancers are present. However, these are guidelines, and cannot identify all whose hereditary risk is increased.

The questionnaires in Appendix A may help you to determine whether you are likely to benefit from Cancer Risk Assessment. Please be aware, however, that not all women who answer "yes" will have an increased risk, and not all of those who answer "no" will not be at increased risk due to hereditary factors.

You may wonder if Cancer Risk Assessment could be useful if your doctor hasn't yet recommended it to you. It's important to realize that doctors and nurses cannot possibly identify everyone who might benefit from Cancer Risk Assessment. Many have a general knowledge of breast cancer risks, but few make it their specialty, have the time to keep up with all the latest developments in this area, or are aware of all whose risk might be increased. Most doctors are busy enough as it is, keeping up with their own areas of expertise and diagnosing and treating illness. Even a superbly informed doctor can rarely devote the number of hours needed to provide a thorough Cancer Risk Assessment. Also, most doctors have never learned how to effectively communicate risk information. In fact, with their focus on medicine and on individuals who have cancer or another illness, physicians and nurses may not be aware of the relief a healthy person or a person who has one or two relatives with cancer can obtain from the Cancer Risk Assessment process.

Because physicians and nurses have less time than they once did in which to take care of their patients' immediate medical needs, often the most pressing issues are the only ones they can cover in the time that is available. This may lead health professionals to overlook the significance of a woman's family history of cancer, particularly if changes occur after the visit in which she and the physician last discussed her family history.

My experience with Candace illustrates how important aspects of a person's family history might be overlooked by physicians, through no fault of theirs or the patient's. Candace came to see me to discuss follow-up options after her diagnosis of atypical hyperplasia. Neither she nor her physician was aware that her breast cancer risk might be increased due to hereditary factors. When Candace's doctor asked if she had relatives with breast cancer, she told him about her father's mother, who was diagnosed with breast cancer "postmenopausally." The presence of this one relative with breast cancer who was diagnosed at an older age did not suggest to her doctor (nor would it even to a geneticist) that there was evidence of an increased hereditary susceptibility to cancer.

When I asked Candace about the health of *each* of her relatives, I learned that her father's sister was diagnosed with ovarian cancer in her early forties. Since her aunt had been diagnosed some years previously and didn't have breast cancer, Candace hadn't thought to mention her aunt's cancer to the doctor. Her doctor may not have realized that the presence of both breast and ovarian cancer can be an indication of increased hereditary cancer risk. Or, the doctor may have thought this type of family history was so rare that it wasn't worth asking all of her patients who had a relative with breast cancer if ovarian cancer was also present in the family. As I can attest, asking about diseases in a person's entire family can be quite time-consuming. The surgeon was taking care of women who needed breast surgery, and so quite logically focused on a family history of breast cancer.

To me, the presence of both breast and ovarian cancer in Candace's family history suggested that strong hereditary factors might well be present. Candace was found to have a BRCA2 mutation, which confirmed that her risk of breast and ovarian cancer was increased. Based on this information, and using the decision-making guidelines in chapter 10, she decided to increase the frequency of her physical breast examinations, to have her yearly mammograms at a nearby breast center, and to have her ovaries removed.

Candace, like many women, initially sought Cancer Risk Assessment to discuss treatment options for atypical hyperplasia, not hereditary cancer risk. Before her first visit with me, she was aware that a woman diagnosed with atypical hyperplasia has a breast cancer risk of less than 1% a year. Candace wanted to talk about the three options she had been given: careful follow-up of her breasts by physical breast examination and mammography; prophylactic mastectomy; and tamoxifen. Since she was perimenopausal, she also had questions about the risks of breast cancer to women with atypical hyperplasia who used hormone replacement therapy. All of these topics are appropriate for Cancer Risk Assessment.

Do remember that your interest and concern are valid reasons for seeking a risk consultation. Not only are there no definitive ways to determine who is and is not at increased risk of cancer, but as you have seen throughout this book, many breast cancer risk factors that are highly touted (such as the reproductive history factors) have little or no meaningful impact on an individual woman's risk. The Cancer Risk Assessment process can therefore be very helpful in terms of the quality of your life, even if you learn that your cancer risks are average.

Of course, you may have been told by a health professional that your cancer risk is high, is increased, or is probably increased due to a family history of cancer or to some other factor. If this is so, even if you are not convinced that your risk may be increased or if you have some anxiety about what you might hear (and the choices you would then make), you would be wise to have your risk checked out in a Cancer Risk Assessment process. *The more you know, the safer you are and the more confident you can be.*

One of my patients, Francine, told me that she put off making an appointment for Cancer Risk Assessment for several years because she feared she would "have to do things I don't want to do" if she were found to be at high risk. She hadn't realized that the process would give her more options, not fewer. With these options comes freedom, including freedom from anxiety. Being afraid, or not learning about what you might do to better safeguard your health, is not freedom and is unlikely to be in your best interest.

Cancer Risk Assessment: Its Structure and Risk Assessment

▨ In the course of Cancer Risk Assessment, you should expect to receive clear, relevant information from a health professional who specializes in cancer risk—whether that person is a geneticist, a physician or a nurse trained in genetics, or a genetic counselor (those with a master's degree in genetic counseling). The substance and depth of the information you receive and *the help you are given in making use of it* are more important than the title of the person providing the service, as suggested by the quote at the beginning of this chapter. Many Cancer Risk Assessment services have started only recently, so the health professional's length of experience in this field is also relevant.

Cancer Risk Assessment can rarely be accomplished in one visit. In my practice, for example, I usually see patients for at least two or three visits. Each visit lasts about one hour. Before the first visit I send a questionnaire covering personal and family history to the woman I will be seeing and then review it with her during the first visit. Whenever possible, I obtain medical records on any of her relatives who were diagnosed with cancer, so that my analysis is based on verified diseases.

Sometimes I find great differences between a relative's disease as noted in the medical reports and what my patient was told about her relative's cancer. For example, my patient may have been told that her grandmother had a stomach or colon cancer, and the records show that she actually had ovarian cancer. Sometimes the records show that a woman's relative who was thought to have breast cancer did not. As you would expect, changes in a relative's diagnosis can greatly influence the risk assessment. I can't always obtain records on a woman's affected relatives, but it is usually worth the effort to attempt to do so. Pathology reports are especially informative. Death certificates, while usually not as accurate or as useful as medical records, may be helpful if the medical records are no longer available.

A relative's medical records sometimes do more than improve the accuracy of the risk analysis. They can also help me to show a woman that the size of her relative's breast cancer was larger than one would expect to find today. Carolyn, whose mother, grandmother, and aunt died of breast cancer, was extremely worried about her own chances of developing and dying of breast cancer. She was certain that in her family all the breast cancers were small when they were found, yet still were fatal. She was amazed—and relieved—when her mother's records showed that she had two cancers in one breast, one 4 cm and the other 3 cm in size. When Carolyn discovered that breast cancers are now far more likely to be found when they are just 1 cm in size or smaller, and learned that her own breasts were not particularly difficult for her doctor to examine or to follow by mammography, she began to feel more confident that she would survive breast cancer if she were diagnosed with it.

Risk Assessment Approaches

☙ Cancer Risk Assessment professionals differ in the methods they use to assess an individual's cancer risk. When you call for an appointment, you may want to ask how the health professional assesses risk and why. In my own practice, I provide information about what is known about each risk factor and use the approaches outlined in chapter 2 for women who have a family history of breast cancer. I do this because, with few exceptions, *we have no reliable scientific data on a woman's overall risk when several factors are present*. The few studies we do have suggest that adding or multiplying a woman's known risks will not produce an accurate overall risk, and will actually overstate an individual's risk.

Given the state of our current information about breast cancer risk, to me it seems more reasonable to use "real life" data than a model. A model is, after all, an unproven intellectual construct for any but the *population* on which it is based. Since we do not yet know how or if different risk factors are combined, I provide the latest information about each risk factor, along with an assessment of the strengths and weaknesses of the studies on which the risks for that factor are based. Some who assess cancer risk have a different philosophy and use two models: The Gail model and the CASH model.[2] I have concerns about the usefulness of both these models in assessing a specific individual's risk.

The Gail Model

The Gail model produces an absolute risk (risk over time in percentages) by using a complex set of equations that *combine* a woman's *relative risks* due to:

- Age,
- Age when her first live child was born,
- Number of breast biopsies,
- Presence of atypical hyperplasia,
- Number of family members with breast cancer (though only mother, sister, or daughter are counted on the maternal side and *no* paternal relatives are included), and
- Race.

There are a number of problems with this approach. First, relative risks are not an accurate way to obtain absolute risks over long periods of time. More important, the Gail model multiplies various relative risks together to obtain one global risk. But, as you saw in chapter 7, women who have a family history of breast cancer do not appear to be at further increased risk when various reproductive history factors are also taken into account.

Third, as you also saw in chapter 7, factors such as a woman's age when she had her first period or when she had her first child actually increase her absolute breast cancer risk very little, if at all. By including a woman's age at the time of her first period and her age when her first child was born as two of the seven items on which overall risk is based, the model assigns far more importance to them than they appear to actually have.

Fourth, this model assumes that a woman's risk rises as the number of her breast biopsies increases. This is too simplistic an approach. In chapter

5 you saw that most benign breast diseases, which sometimes but not always lead to a biopsy, either do not increase absolute breast cancer risk or do so only slightly. Fifth, the model counts how many of a woman's close relatives have had breast cancer (which is also simplistic), but then does not include *all* the relevant relatives. For example, it ignores all grandparents and aunts and all paternal history.

The Gail model tends to *overestimate* risk, particularly risk to young women. In one large study of nurses, for example, the model overpredicted breast cancer risk by 33% to the study group as a whole.[3] For women younger than age 50 or who had a first child before age 20, there was a twofold overestimation of risk. To their credit, the developers of the model have urged caution in applying it. Even if a good fit were to be found between this model and a group of women, it would not lend credibility to the model's ability to assess an *individual's* risk. It would instead demonstrate that the model could estimate risk in that population. Individual and population risks should not be confused.

Many clinicians find that the Gail model is a quick and easy way to come up with an estimate of an individual woman's breast cancer risk and either don't realize its basic shortcomings or are not concerned about them. Some say that although the Gail model is not accurate, "It's all we've got." My own feeling is that it is better to acknowledge that we don't currently know enough to be able to usefully combine risks due to different factors than to give the impression that the Gail model can provide a woman with a useful estimate of her risk.

Unfortunately, the Gail model, developed by statisticians to approximate risks in populations, is now being widely used to determine an individual woman's risk. Many physicians were sent a computer disk or hand calculator by pharmaceutical companies to enable them to "simply" and "easily" assess their patients' breast cancer risks. By entering into the computer the number of biopsies a woman has had, the number of affected relatives, race, and other factors that I listed above, a physician can get a quick result about a woman's risk for the next five years or up to her nineties. Most health professionals are not statisticians, so many of them undoubtedly have more confidence in the risks a computer program or calculator generates than they would if they knew the model's shortcomings. If the health professional you contact uses only the Gail model to assess breast cancer risk, I suggest you keep looking.

The CASH Model

To assess risk due to a family history of breast cancer, many who provide Cancer Risk Assessment use what has come to be called the CASH model, since it was based on data collected in the Cancer and Steroid Hormone study. I am uneasy using the CASH model approach to assess family history risk for several reasons. First, the model was developed from a population of women who had various types of family histories. The number who had a mother or sister with breast cancer was large, but for many other family history types few women were available to be included in the groups on which risks were calculated. Risks based on small numbers of individuals are less likely to be accurate than those that are larger.

Second, a number of studies have shown (as discussed in chapter 2), that individuals with similar-appearing family histories can have very different risks. Third, this is only a model, which means that the risks are based on a number of unproven assumptions. As with the Gail model, I feel that in making risk assessments it is more prudent to use information based on actual study populations.

In my own assessments of risk due to family history I tend to use the studies described in chapter 2, some of which were conducted by individuals who later developed the CASH model. When I use these studies I tell my patients about the possible effects of heterogeneity. I also, of course, make use of results from studies of women who have BRCA mutations, again keeping heterogeneity in mind.

I believe that this is a time for health professionals who assess cancer risk to fully disclose all that we *do not* know and to help the people we see to understand why the risks are likely to change as more is learned. A realization of the limits of current information is as important as information about the risk of developing cancer, and the chances of finding a cancer before it is life threatening. The point of a risk assessment is, after all, not just the risk that is obtained but what a person can do about it.

Cancer Risk Assessment: Using the Information

❧ Risk assessment is part, but not all, of the important information individuals should expect to obtain in a Cancer Risk Assessment service. To be most useful, a discussion of the origin of cancer, survival rates for breast and other cancers, and help in decision making should always be included in this service, since its aim is to increase the quantity and improve the quality of an individual's life.

Women who seek Cancer Risk Assessment need sufficient time to process the often sophisticated and potentially unsettling information they may receive. Feelings about risk and one's own vulnerability to cancer generally change with time and with increased understanding, so time must be made available for these changes in perspective to occur. In addition to information about cancer risk, women often obtain the following from Cancer Risk Assessment:

- Information to help develop a useful and safe breast health or treatment plan
- A freeing up of energy that often results when a person feels that she can make reasonable decisions based on sufficient information
- Information about cancer risks to one's relatives so they also can institute appropriate follow-up
- Information about how cancer develops, which in turn generally leads to demystifying cancer and an increased peace of mind
- Assistance in living more comfortably with uncertainty

Making use of cancer risk information and learning to live with uncertainty are so important that I have devoted chapters 10 and 11 to a discussion of these topics.

Genetic Testing

Genetic testing for hereditary cancer risk is sometimes, but not always, useful in the Cancer Risk Assessment process. Many people benefit without being tested. In making a decision about whether to have genetic testing, individuals generally weigh the following:

- Cost
- Probability of finding a mutation that increases cancer risk
- Likelihood that a definitive test result would:
    - Enhance the quality of life

- Lead to a change in health and/or medical care
- Enhance a relative's quality of life or lead a relative to change her health and/or medical care.

I'll discuss each of these in turn.

Cost

In 2000, the fee to test for all known BRCA mutations was over $2,500. Once a mutation was detected in a family, the fee for testing other family members was about $300. The cost of testing for the three mutations most often found in individuals of Ashkenazi Jewish descent was about $400. These costs do deter some from genetic testing if insurance coverage is not available. For example, Carol, who was 38, had concerns about her risk due to a family history of cancer. Her mother and maternal aunt were diagnosed with breast cancer in their forties and her maternal grandmother with ovarian cancer in her sixties. Carol's aunt was alive, but her mother and grandmother had died. Ideally, then, the person to test first in Carol's family was her aunt. After several family discussions, with much concern expressed about the possibility that more than $2,500 might be spent without finding a mutation in Carol's aunt, the family decided not to pursue genetic testing.

Instead, Carol decided that she would continue to have her breasts carefully checked and would have her ovaries removed. She said, "Even if my aunt and I test positive, I won't have my breasts removed. And even if my aunt has a mutation and I test negative, I'll still worry about my risk of ovarian cancer. Since I've had my kids, I think I'll spend the money on ovarian surgery instead of testing." Carol had her ovaries removed laparoscopically, continued to take birth control pills as a way of maintaining her hormone levels, and says she feels fine.

Insurance Coverage

Several large insurance companies and HMOs have developed guidelines for determining when they will pay for genetic testing. Other groups are likely to follow. Some of my patients are concerned about telling their insurance companies that they are seeking genetic testing for fear that their ability to obtain medical, life, and disability insurance may be limited in the future if they are found to carry a mutation.

There have actually been very few documented instances of medical insurance discrimination—or any other type, despite the amount of media attention devoted to this issue. According to a recent study reported in the *Journal of the American Medical Association,* "little or no indication of discriminatory policies or practices by insurers based on genetic test information" was found.[4] Increasingly, laws are being passed on national and state levels to protect people from what is called "genetic discrimination."

Some of the large insurance companies have even agreed to pay for testing without seeking to learn the results. Still, at a time when health insurance companies and medical coverage are both in a state of volatile change, it is not surprising to me that some of my patients who seek genetic testing pay for the test themselves and do not go through their insurance company. This is an area of great worry to many people, but one that is likely to subside as new laws are passed and testing is more widespread.

Likelihood That Mutation Is Present

In chapter 4, I discussed the increased risk of breast and ovarian cancer to women who carry a BRCA mutation and presented information about families in which a mutation is more likely to be found—for example, families in which an individual was diagnosed with both breast and ovarian cancer. Based on your concern and your ability to pay for testing, you can use these probabilities to decide whether testing makes sense in your situation. For example, if there is a 5% chance that a mutation will be found, are you interested in testing? What about a 15% chance or a 40% chance? Remember also that even if a geneticist thinks that your family history shows *no* evidence of an increased hereditary risk, this assessment is no guarantee. A mutation could still be found, but is unlikely to be present.

The reverse is also possible. You may have many relatives with breast and other cancers, but no mutation will be found in the family. In this case, you still could have an increased hereditary cancer risk due to mutations that scientists cannot currently find. The point is that assessment of family history cannot provide definitive information about which individuals or families will carry a mutation that can be detected with current genetic-testing techniques. Such an assessment can only tell you the likelihood. Also, as you saw in chapter 4, a negative test result cannot always assure a woman that her hereditary cancer risk is not increased. Due to these uncertainties, it is particularly important for you to participate in the decision-making process.

When Knowing the Result Would Really Matter

People are more likely to seek genetic testing if the results will change how they view themselves in the world or the way in which they or a relative will proceed with their health and medical care. A woman who feels anxious or "doomed" by her family history may have testing to learn whether this foreboding is actually so for her or not. If she does not carry the mutation that was found in her family, a great load of worry will generally be removed from her life. If she is found to carry the mutation, she knows that her concerns are well founded and that she needs to carefully think through the follow-up and treatment options that are best suited for her. I present guidelines about how to do this in chapter 10.

In my own practice I find that women who have a concern about breast cancer risk and not their risk of ovarian cancer may decide not to have genetic testing. They say that knowing the test results will not lead them to change their already rigorous breast health program. Others, who feel that it would be difficult to find a small cancer in their breasts, choose testing. These women say that if they are found to have a mutation they will have prophylactic mastectomies. If they do not carry a mutation they will not have the surgery—even though they realize that a mutation that increases breast cancer risk might be present.

Concerns about ovarian cancer risk lead the women I see to seek testing far more often than do their concerns about breast cancer risk. As I discuss in chapter 10, most ovarian cancers have spread by the time they are found. The five-year survival rate is about 44%. To reduce their chances of developing ovarian cancer, women at increased risk generally consider having their ovaries removed. Those who learn that they are mutation carriers often have their ovaries removed, while the others, the non-carriers, usually do not. When test results are not informative I find that many women also choose to have their ovaries removed. Testing can therefore play an important role in helping women make this important decision, and may help some women to avoid surgery or to feel better about having it.

The results of genetic testing need to be interpreted with caution, as you saw in chapter 4. In some instances these results may not be as clear-cut as a woman assumes they will be. For example, Ellen was a 54-year-old woman whose mother had been diagnosed with ovarian cancer in her forties. One of her mother's sisters was diagnosed with breast cancer in her fifties. Ellen wanted genetic testing for two reasons: to provide information that might be helpful to other people in the family who had not been diagnosed with cancer, and to see if she was at increased risk of breast and ovarian cancer herself. When we first met she said: "If I have a mutation I'll know my risk of ovarian cancer is high and I'll have my ovaries removed. If I don't have a mutation I won't need to worry about it."

Before Ellen was tested, I explained that since none of her affected relatives was alive, the test result could not be interpreted so simply. If she were tested and found not to carry a mutation, she could still have an increased risk of breast and ovarian cancer due to mutations that can't be detected at present. As you may remember from chapter 4, genetic testing can detect most but not all mutations in the BRCA genes. And this test can detect none of the mutations in other genes that also might increase breast and ovarian cancer risk. Therefore, without finding a mutation in a close relative, a negative test result for her would be noninformative. In this case Ellen decided to proceed with testing. She could afford the fee of over $2,000 and felt it would be money well spent, even if she were to have a negative (noninformative) result. Ellen's test result was positive, however, which meant she had inherited a mutation that increased her risk of breast and ovarian cancer. Needless to say, Ellen was pleased that her decision provided useful information. She had her ovaries removed and says she feels "lighter and more free" than before.

Once a BRCA mutation had been identified in Ellen, it was possible for her brothers, sisters, cousins, and children to be tested as well. Ellen's oldest child was a daughter of 24 who said she thought she would wait several years before being tested. Two of Ellen's siblings were also found to carry the mutations, as were three of her cousins. "I felt that I was giving a big present to the whole family," she said. "Now that they know what their risks are they can be better protected."

As I hope these examples demonstrate, no one can decide for another how important the test results will be. A woman who has not been diagnosed with cancer and who has no living close relative with cancer may decide to proceed with testing. Sometimes a mutation is found, showing that her risk of breast and ovarian cancer is increased. Or a woman who has a strong family history of cancer but who has no living affected relative may be tested and no mutation will be found. In this case the negative test result is not informative and does not necessarily mean that a mutation that increases cancer risk is not present, only that none has been found. Without a close relative who is found to carry a mutation, there is no way to distinguish between these possibilities.

For some, the cost of testing will be more burdensome than to others, so women who can afford it are more likely to request testing than women who can't, even when the chance of finding a BRCA mutation is small or if a negative result will be uninformative. Sometimes a family will come together to contribute funds to help the first individual in the family be tested. If a mutation is found in that person, future testing for others in the family will be less expensive since the testing will be for that single mutation only.

Living with Genetic Test Results

Women's reactions to test results differ, as might be expected. What follows is a sampling of some of the more frequent reactions that I encounter.

Shock

Women who choose testing usually do so because they feel that they have a high cancer risk. When a woman finds that she does *not* carry a mutation and does *not* have an increased hereditary risk of cancer, she may experience a sense of shock, say she is numb, and may even ask if the testing laboratory has made a mistake. (While a mistake is theoretically possible, it is extremely unlikely with a reputable laboratory that does testing of this sort on a regular basis.) Others are surprised to find that they don't feel an immediate sense of relief and release. They usually *will* feel less anxious, but time may be needed before they can fully accept the result emotionally. After all, many of these women say they had "felt in their bones" that they would be diagnosed with cancer one day. Now, with the test result, they are being asked to see themselves as having the average woman's risk, or at least not having the high risk of a mutation carrier. This dramatic change in a person's sense of self can take time.

Guilt

Some women who find that they didn't inherit the family mutation wonder how they "deserve" to be so lucky. Some feel guilt—sometimes called survivor guilt—at being spared. Some don't understand how they could possibly *not* have the mutation carried by a relative since they so closely resemble her. The answer is, of course, that many genes (and the environment in which a person is raised) contribute to similarities with a relative. An increased hereditary risk of breast cancer is primarily due to a change in only one single gene.

Worry

Women who learn that they do not carry the family mutation some-times worry about how to tell their brothers and sisters who were found to be mutation carriers. They are concerned about hurting their relatives' feelings, fear that their siblings will feel jealous, and sometimes have a sense of being an outsider in their family. Children of mutation carriers who test negative often say they can't wait to let Mom or Dad "off the hook" and add that their parent's worry about them will now decrease.

Denial

Sometimes people forget the uninformative nature of a negative result in the first person in the family who is tested. This happened in Deborah's family. Her mother, grandmother, and aunt had all been diagnosed with breast cancer. Her mother was the first affected person in the family to be tested, and no mutation was found. When I told Deborah's mother about the negative finding, her first reaction was, "Oh, thank goodness. I'm so glad I didn't pass on anything bad to Deborah." I reminded Deborah's mother that her family history was one in which an increased risk of can-cer due to hereditary factors was probably present, whether current tech-nology could detect a mutation in her or not. Since no mutation was found, it would not now be possible to test Deborah to see if her risk of cancer was increased. In this case, the finding of no mutation was *not* good news. Deborah's mother knew all this but had momentarily forgotten. She realized intellectually that her daughter could inherit a mutation that in-creased cancer risk from her, but, like most parents, emotionally shrank from the idea that she carried a mutation that could increase her children's risk of cancer.

Relief and Uncertainty

Women who were diagnosed with breast cancer often seek testing to try to learn whether their risk of ovarian cancer is increased. These women are concerned about their ovarian cancer risk, but are reluctant to have their ovaries removed without more definitive information than can be provided by a family history assessment. Often in these instances the women have no cases of ovarian cancer in their family, only breast cancer. Those in whom a mutation is found are generally quite relieved and say, "Now I know that removing my ovaries is what I need to do." They are also pleased that informative testing is now available for their relatives.

Women who have been diagnosed with breast cancer and who are not found to carry a mutation often face a more complex decision-making process, especially if no ovarian cancer is present in the family. This is because assessment of family history by itself cannot definitively rule out that a woman's risk of ovarian cancer is not increased, so they may be left with a nagging worry. Some, but not all of these women, also decide to have their ovaries removed, particularly if they are postmenopausal or have completed their families.

Taking Charge

Women without a cancer diagnosis in whom a mutation is found often accept the finding quickly, saying, "I knew the result before I had the test." Or "I've always felt I was at high risk." There may also be tears, fear, and a sense of regret, of course. However, most quickly begin making plans and take action. These women generally institute an intense round of visits to physicians to determine what their follow-up and treatment will be. Some worry that their relatives who do not carry a mutation will be overly concerned about their ability to cope with the test results. These women often tell me that their relatives don't realize how fortunate they, the mutation carriers, feel to have had access to testing, to early detection, and to treatment options that were not available previously. Many say that the test results have taken them out of limbo and given them the energy and incentive to move ahead with their lives.

These are just brief examples. Each individual has a different personality and each family a different dynamic, and both of these factors influence reactions to test results. Some of the greatest difficulties women report come from what they perceive as the "overreaction" of those around them, including that of some physicians. Genetic testing is new, so many doctors have little or no experience with either testing results or the "high risk" status of women with a mutation. If you, a friend, or relative is tested, be sure that you or she receives enough information to make reasonable, realistic plans and are given the time to do this. You will not be helped if you are treated as an endangered person because your risks are now known to be increased, nor are you likely to benefit if you are undertreated *or* overtreated by a health professional who has little experience with genetic testing. (To help you more effectively navigate the medical system, you may want to reread chapter 8.) Cancer Risk Assessment may be of particular help to you also, since the health professionals who provide this service are likely to have experience with women who are called "high risk" or who carry a BRCA mutation.

Key Points to Remember

- Assessment of cancer risk is most effectively provided by a health professional with special training in cancer genetics. This person may be a geneticist; a physician or nurse trained in genetics; or a genetic counselor.
- If you are afraid of hearing "bad news" about your cancer risk, please bear in mind that living with a nagging worry or concern and without an effective health plan is not useful.
- Cancer Risk Assessment may be especially beneficial if you:
  - Have a family history of cancer or have been diagnosed with cancer
  - Have been diagnosed with benign breast disease, ductal carcinoma in situ, or lobular carcinoma in situ
  - Have concerns about risk due to hormone replacement therapy, birth control pills, or some other factor in your environment
  - Have questions about reproductive factors, such as not having given birth to a child
  - Would like help in making decisions about your breast health care or treatment.
- It is perfectly reasonable to go for Cancer Risk Assessment if you have questions or concerns about your cancer risk, even if your physician has not suggested that you do so or is not concerned about your risk. You cannot assume that your physician will have the latest information about cancer risk, since this is not his or her area of expertise.

- In seeking a Cancer Risk Assessment, look for a provider who assesses risks based on available studies and does not rely on computer programs, models, or composite risks.
- In the Cancer Risk Assessment process, expect to discuss your individual risks, a follow-up plan, survival rates, the latest treatment options, your relatives' potential risks, and the origins of cancer.
- If you receive some unsettling or surprising information during Cancer Risk Assessment, *take time to process it* before making any important decisions. You may want to schedule several visits with specialists of different types to be clear about the issues.
- With genetic testing, proper *interpretation* of results is as important as the results themselves. For instance, a mutation may *not* be found, but you may have an increased risk due to hereditary factors. Or a mutation may be found, putting you at a higher risk of developing cancer, but this does not mean that you will ever develop cancer. It is important to discuss your risk factors and test results with someone trained in cancer genetics.
- Genetic testing is one of the tools used in Cancer Risk Assessment, not the only reason for using this service. Testing is most likely to be useful to you if the information you obtain will:
  - Enhance the quality of your life
  - Change how you will proceed with your health and medical care.

Elements of Informed Decision Making

Decisions about personal risks require, at a minimum, information about the nature and likelihood of potential ill effects,
information about the risk factors that modify one's susceptibility, and information about the ease or difficulty of avoiding
harm.[1]

We hear a lot these days about a woman's need to make "informed decisions" about her health and medical care. Unfortunately this sometimes
means that she is asked to rather quickly choose between several options
after hearing briefly about each one. In these instances, her decision may
not be truly informed, but instead may be largely determined by what she
has heard in the past and what she thinks a trusted medical authority be-
lieves is best for her. This approach does not lead to what I would call informed decision making, since the individual has not learned enough to be
able to realistically weigh the pros and cons of each option before choosing what will work best for her.

Informed decisions are, of course, a very personal matter. No two
people are alike, nor do any two people go about making decisions in the
same way. Your level of concern about breast or ovarian cancer may be
lower than another woman's. Or you may have a lower tolerance for
uncertainty than another equally responsible person. And, of course,
lifestyles and value systems vary among people. All of these can lead to different—but equally valid—decisions for women who have the same risks.

In this chapter I discuss guidelines and elements for you to consider in making decisions about the use of early detection modalities and the methods that are sometimes suggested as ways to prevent breast and ovarian cancer. As you read this chapter, it is important to focus on what makes the most sense to *you*. People differ. Just as no one car, vacation, or movie suits all, so no one breast health program is for all who have the same risk factors. With regard to breast and ovarian health care, the main person to please is yourself. Once you have information about a technique or procedure, once you have considered the options and have given yourself time to reflect, follow through on what feels right for you, even if it is different from what might be recommended for the "average woman" or "high-risk woman"—whoever they are!

To make an informed and realistic decision about breast health care, you will need:

1. Information about your risk of developing breast cancer

2. Information about the likely prognosis if you should be diagnosed with breast cancer

3. Help in recognizing and moving through emotions that might act as barriers to your understanding or ability to take appropriate action

4. Information about the efficacy of early detection techniques and measures that are said to be preventive

The first points were covered in earlier chapters. In this chapter I focus on the last point—making decisions about early detection techniques and "preventive" approaches.

Mammography

In 1999 the American Cancer Society mammography guidelines called for women to have yearly mammograms beginning at age 40. Other groups also recommend that women start mammograms at 40, but suggest a mammogram "every one to two years" from 40 to 49, with yearly mammograms beginning at age 50. The difference in recommendations appears to be due to how groups weigh the results of studies in which women were found to derive little or no benefit by having mammography in their forties. The results of these studies are difficult to interpret, particularly since fewer breast cancers are found in younger than in older women. Also, younger women are more likely to have denser breast tissue than older women, making it more difficult for mammography to detect a breast cancer in younger women than those who are older.

Because women in their forties develop fewer breast cancers than older women, interpretation of results can be hampered by the smaller numbers of breast cancers that are available to analyze in this group. Also, years must pass before a survival benefit resulting from mammography can be seen. Improved methodology also needs to be taken into account. In the last fifteen years mammography equipment, films, and techniques have improved significantly. For example, mammography technologists now regularly take courses that include topics such as the positioning of the breast to include as much of the breast for examination as possible. At the same time, radiologists (the physicians who read mammograms) have become increasingly better trained in detecting small breast cancers. For these reasons, a woman's breast cancer is more likely to be detected currently than would a similar cancer some years ago.

One recent study confirmed previous findings about the life-saving benefits of yearly mammography for women age 50 and older.[2] It also showed in a most elegant fashion that younger women, whose breast cancers tend to be faster-growing, can pass more rapidly through the "non-palpable" (unable to be felt) stage. For younger women there is *less* time during which breast cancers can be picked up by mammography before they grow to a size that can be felt.

Based on their data, the authors estimate that for women aged 40 to 49 a breast cancer takes an average of 2.5 years to grow from the time it could be detected on a mammogram to the time it can first be felt in a physical examination. For women age 50 to 59 an average of 3.8 years is needed for this growth to occur and for women 60 to 69 it takes 4.3 years. The results of this study suggest that as a group younger women would benefit *more* from yearly mammograms than older women, since younger women's breast cancers can pass more rapidly from the time their cancers can be seen on a mammogram to when they can be felt. Because younger women are more likely to have faster-growing tumors, more frequent mammograms appear to make good sense in this group. The authors conclude that if mammography is to help save the lives of women aged 40 to 49, they must have it every 12 to 18 months.

In a study of over one thousand women age 35 and younger, mammography was not found to be useful to the 23 women who were diagnosed with breast cancer in this age group.[3] In these young women, all of the cancers were felt before they had a mammogram. Of course, very, very few women are diagnosed with breast cancer before age 35, and almost none in this age group have regular mammograms, partly because the risk of breast cancer is so low and partly because these women tend to have dense breast tissue, which makes mammographic detection of breast cancer exceedingly difficult.

Women who have a strong family history of breast cancer or who are concerned about their breast cancer risk for other reasons may choose to start their mammograms before age 40, even though current studies show no benefit. Some clinicians recommend starting mammography ten years before the earliest diagnosis of breast cancer in a woman's family. There is no scientific evidence to suggest that this is the best way to proceed, however.

If you decide to have a mammogram before age 40, as many of my patients with a strong family history of breast cancer do, you should remember that mammograms do not find all breast cancers, particularly in younger women. For this reason, physical breast examinations are also very important. Unfortunately, I find that many women neglect physical breast examinations and instead focus only on their mammogram. Some also fail to realize how important it is to have a mammogram yearly and to make prior films available to the radiologist to compare with those taken most recently.

Physical Breast Examinations

Physical breast examinations can play an important role in finding breast cancers—whether you do them yourself or have them done by a health professional. The 1999 American Cancer Society guidelines for physical breast suggest that:

- Women 20 years and older examine their own breasts monthly.
- Women age 20 to 39 have a physical breast examination by a doctor or nurse every three years.

- Women 40 and older have a physical breast examination by a doctor or nurse every year.

Lack of Regular Physical Breast Examinations

☙ Many women tell me it is all they can do to get up their courage to have a yearly mammogram and that they do little beyond this for their breast health care. They either don't examine their own breasts, do so in a cursory or sporadic manner, or have at most one breast examination a year by a health professional. Neglecting regular breast self-examinations (BSE) and examinations by a health professional can be unwise, since many breast lumps are found first by physical examination and not on a mammogram. It is the combination of mammography and physical breast examination that provides a woman the best guarantee that a breast cancer will be found at the earliest possible stage.

Some of you may feel that your concern about breast cancer is so high that if you were to examine your breasts you might deny the presence of any breast lump you felt. As Marcie said:

> Any time I examine myself I have to face the questions of whether there's something going on. And it's almost like I can't even ask myself that question. So I may examine myself and I'll feel something and I'll get anxious and say to myself, well, I know I'm anxious anyway so how do I know what I feel?

Perhaps you have decided not to examine your breasts because you might imagine a lump was there when it wasn't. Ruth told me, "I hate to be worried about my own body. I have an active imagination and I will imagine something is there." Or, like Janice, you may feel your breasts are too difficult for you to examine.

Some women avoid BSE because they are unsure what they would or could do if they found a lump or thickening. As Janice said:

> If you check your breasts and there is a lump you have to do something about it. If you don't check your breasts and you don't know, you don't have to do anything.

You may avoid BSE because you fear that in the process your anxiety will increase: "When I try to do a breast exam I get more anxious because then I get more caught up in it again and the emotionality and worry come up again."

Or, as Marsha said:

> I don't want that responsibility for myself. I don't want to have
> to fool around and wonder if this is a new lump or an old lump,
> is it a cancer or not. I don't want to have to deal with that. It's
> pretty babyish but that's how I feel about it.

If you feel this way, instead of walking around and figuratively "beating yourself on the breast" for not taking better care of yourself, there *is* another way! First, you can ask for personal instruction in this technique. Many physicians, nurses, and nurse practitioners now offer quite useful personal instruction in BSE. Having a "hands on" lesson often helps a woman to feel more comfortable about examining her own breasts.

One woman told me that for her, reading a pamphlet about how to do BSE was like trying to learn how to ride a bicycle by looking at a few diagrams. So, don't feel that you should be able to examine your breasts with confidence just by reading about it. Sometimes personal instruction can make all the difference. Who, after all, expects to be able to play tennis after reading a pamphlet?

Like many women who have a concern about breast cancer risk, you may well find that your anxiety is reduced and your sense of peace and security is increased by having a health professional examine your breasts every four to six months. Remember, very few breast cancers grow from non-palpable to larger than 1 cm (a little less than half an inch) in four months. As you may remember from chapter 2, recent studies show breast cancer survival rates of better than 90% all the way to twenty years for most women with small breast cancers.[4] Therefore, regular physical breast examinations by a health professional in conjunction with a yearly mammogram can increase the chance that if you should develop breast cancer, it would be found before it is life threatening.

If you learn that your breast cancer risk is lower than you expected, whether through risk analysis or with genetic testing, you may need some time to adjust to this new lower risk and new view of yourself. Understandably, you may find yourself reluctant to scale back to the average woman's follow-up schedule. Because of your past experiences with cancer, you may be determined to do everything you can to ensure early detection—and then some. In fact, you may choose a more rigorous follow-up program than your health professional feels is necessary. That's entirely up to you. You are the expert about your life and what you need to help you live more comfortably. For example, many of the women I see who are or who feel that they are at high risk see a health professional every four months for a breast examination.

From my perspective, your peace of mind is as good a guide as any to use in setting up a physical breast examination schedule. After all, you have your concerns for a reason. You deserve to be treated by a capable, understanding doctor or nurse who will see you promptly when you have a breast concern and who will be respectful of your needs for vigilant follow-up breast care. (Do be aware that most radiologists do not recommend routine mammography more than once a year.)

Prophylactic Mastectomy

ℜ Many women shrink from even thinking about having their breasts removed before a cancer diagnosis (prophylactic mastectomy). Others tell me, "I just want to have them off so I can get on with my life. I don't want to always be thinking about breast cancer." Still others say, "Deciding to have my breasts removed was one of the hardest things in my life. I tell people to think long and hard before they do it. It's rough." Yet others tell me in no uncertain terms, "I was so relieved to have them gone. It's been no big deal for me."

Here, too, as you can see, women differ. What is right for one won't work for another. If you are considering prophylactic mastectomy, it's important to be sure that you do all you can to be sure that this approach is what you want and need.

Unfortunately, many women who choose prophylactic mastectomy are not satisfied with their choice, even years later. Of nearly 600 women who were asked about their surgeries an average of fourteen years later, 20% said they were dissatisfied and 25% said they felt less feminine. More than a quarter reported that their cancer fears had not lessened after surgery.[5]

Women are more likely to be comfortable with their decision to have pro-phylactic mastectomy if they received help in thinking through the risks and benefits beforehand and if they were the ones to initially suggest it, ac-cording to a study in which most of the women were satisfied with their surgeries.[6]

The value of prophylactic mastectomy, the removal of a woman's breasts to reduce her chances of developing breast cancer, has been de-bated in medical circles for years. This is a difficult area in which to do a study, since no one knows who will or won't be diagnosed with breast cancer. One recent study of women with a family history of breast cancer who had prophylactic mastectomy reported a "reduction in the incidence of breast cancer of at least 90%."[7] As you can imagine, this report raised quite a stir. Who wouldn't want to reduce her breast cancer risk by such a "great amount"? You may have noticed that the result was reported as a 90% reduction. The next question is, of course, "90% less *than what?*" Once again, I think you will be surprised by the small number of breast cancers involved. *If you accept this study's assumptions and risk assessment approaches,* 621 women underwent prophylactic mastectomy to save 18 lives. Of the women in the study who were estimated to have a moderately increased risk, 98% were not helped by prophylactic mas-tectomy.

The study estimated a woman's chance of developing breast cancer by using two methods: family history assessment and the Gail model. I have already shown in chapters 2 and 9 how inexact both these approaches can be. Family history assessment is inexact since women with apparently similar family histories can have cancers due to different causes and so have very different risks. The Gail model is generally *not* used to estimate risk when a family history of cancer is present, since it does not take pa-ternal family history into account and uses crude methods to assign risk, based on only some maternal relatives. You may remember that the Gail model tends to inflate risk, and so is likely to overestimate the number of expected breast cancers. A high number of expected cancers would, in turn, inflate the number of breast cancers "prevented" by prophylactic mastectomy.

For example, suppose you wanted to know how successful an insecti-cide was in preventing beetles from eating a plant. If you estimated that beetles would have eaten two tons without insecticide use and found that they ate only one ton when insecticides were used, you would have a 50% crop loss. However, if you estimated that the beetles would have eaten ten tons and they ate only one ton when insecticides were used, you would have a 10% loss. In both cases the beetles ate one ton. By changing the estimated amount that they *might* have eaten, you will obtain different amounts of loss. The same approach was used in the prophylactic mastectomy study. Just as no one knows how much the beetles *might* have eaten, no one knows how many cancers might have occurred.

This study used breast cancer mortality data from 1973 to 1992. Its findings about lives saved due to prophylactic mastectomy, don't apply to women diagnosed in the late 1990s and beyond, since breast cancer prognosis is now greatly improved. Therefore, the use of mortality rates from 1973 to 1992 will inflate the chance of death due to breast cancer in a woman diagnosed with breast cancer today. The study estimated that 18 lives would be saved by removing the breasts of over 600 women. Because far fewer women now die of breast cancer than were likely to do so in the years of the study, it is clear that fewer than 18 lives would be saved today, even if you accept this study's flawed premise. Careful assessment of this study shows that its results do not support a clear or large benefit of prophylactic mastectomy to women diagnosed with breast cancer today.

Because of the excellent prognosis of women whose breast cancers are found at a small size, modern informed decision making about prophylactic mastectomy is complete only if it encompasses more than information about a woman's breast cancer risk. In addition, the ease or chance of detecting a small cancer in a woman's breasts must be taken into account. Also, women who undergo prophylactic mastectomy need to be aware that all breast tissue cannot be removed, so cancer could still occur in the breast area.

At this point you, like many of my patients, may want to ask me what I would do if I were in your shoes, or if you were my mother, daughter, or sister. I can honestly say that I don't know what I would do in such a circumstance, since I am not currently in it. Unless I were you right now, I couldn't know what I would do. The point is, of course, to determine for yourself what feels right for *you* right now.

If you were my patient, I would help you to evaluate the situation to see if you appear to:

- Be heading in a direction that seems to fit you.
- Have heard enough of the information about your risks and the ease of detecting cancer in your breast for the information to begin to make sense both intellectually and emotionally.
- Have had time to process new information.
- Be making decisions to please yourself, not others.

Sometimes my patients make decisions that surprise me. Their decision may be right for them, even if it puzzles me. When someone makes a decision that doesn't appear congruent to me, and I have communicated this to my patient, I remind myself that I am hearing only part of a complex decision-making process, and that this partial information can skew my viewpoint. The person making the decision is her own best expert—once she has the most up-to-date information and an opportunity to make up her own mind. In the same way, if you should be making this decision and a dear friend or relative does not agree with you, the decision you make may still be the right one for you. This is an important point, since it is sometimes tempting to look to others at this emotional time instead of appreciating that individuals are best served in the long run by trusting themselves to make the decisions that are best for them.

On the other hand, as Tanya's experience demonstrates, a dear one's doubts and concern are sometimes crucial in helping a woman arrive at the decision that is right for her. When I first saw Tanya she was scheduled to have both breasts removed in two weeks, since she had recently been diagnosed with atypical hyperplasia. She said, "I know me. I can't live comfortably with such a high risk. I know I will worry all the time." I was unaware of her planned surgery, or I would not have seen her for a first visit so close to its scheduled date. At the beginning of the visit she announced: "I'm just here because my surgeon and my husband keep badgering me to talk to you. I've already made up my mind to have surgery. This visit is to make them happy."

When I reviewed general risk information with Tanya, she began to have doubts about the magnitude of her risk. She became angry, started to shake, cried, and said that I was "mixing her up for nothing." She and her husband began to argue, and continued to do so up to the end of the visit.

To Tanya's credit, and that of her husband, she postponed surgery and kept her next appointment with me. We again reviewed her breast cancer risks and the pros and cons of surgery. She and her husband said they had been arguing all week. Tanya eventually decided not to have her breasts removed. "My risks are far lower than I could have believed," she said. She later sent me flowers and a note of appreciation for "hanging in there with her."

When I saw Tanya and her husband several years later, she expressed gratitude for her husband's strong stance. He replied by explaining that at the time Tanya was planning to have her prophylactic mastectomies he wasn't against the surgery, since he was unsure about what her risks actually were. He was sure, however, that prior to his wife's first visit with me, she had made the decision for surgery in a way that was not characteristic of her and that was not comfortable for him. "I saw trouble down the road with all this racing ahead," he said.

As with Tanya, whenever possible, I try to slow down an action that seems precipitous or not clearly thought through. This can be particularly important if, as discussed in chapter 8, a woman received an "imprint" of fear from an interaction with a doctor she saw during a time of stress. In Tanya's case, she felt caught between the *feeling* that she was at greatly increased risk and *new information* suggesting that her risks were far less than she initially believed. The dissonance between the two led to her emotional distress. She needed time to process the new information so the emotional and the intellectual aspects could became congruent.

Lorraine was another woman who felt caught between new information and prior imprinting. When I discussed risk with her, she became quite agitated, saying that what I was telling her couldn't be so since it differed from what her doctor had told her. As her anxiety increased, she began to interrupt, angrily contradicting her husband and me each time we started to speak. I then stopped, thought a bit, and told Lorraine that I didn't think I could help her that day. I explained that the information I was giving her seemed to be at variance with her beliefs and that I didn't want to challenge them. I told her I thought I had useful information, but it wouldn't help someone who didn't want to hear it. As a result, we weren't getting anywhere. I was therefore ending the session early and would not charge her for it.

To my amazement, Lorraine responded by declaring that she wasn't going to leave. Clearly she was very upset. I responded by saying that I would continue the session if she could accept that I was trying to help and was on her side. My job was to help her hear new information about a topic she had considered closed. I acknowledged that it was obviously frustrating and discouraging for her to hear information that differed from what she had previously heard and accepted. I concluded by assuring her that if we worked together and not apart, she could certainly stay.

From that time on, the sessions went well. When Lorraine checked with her doctor she was amazed to discover that he had no disagreement with my risk assessment. She had overinterpreted some of the cautions her doctor was trying to express. Lorraine later expressed her thanks to me. I tell her story to demonstrate how deeply touched and concerned individuals can be at this time. Some act in an angry, combative fashion, when they are actually frightened.

Connie, another patient with a family history of breast cancer, surprised me by saying that her surgeon had urged her, in the strongest terms, to consider prophylactic mastectomy. I knew her surgeon as someone who rarely recommended prophylactic mastectomy and so asked Connie if I could call her doctor to discuss the case. Connie was delighted to have me do so. When I called the surgeon, she said that Connie had expressed so much anxiety over so many visits that she was unsure any course other than prophylactic mastectomy would meet her emotional needs. According to the surgeon, from the time prophylactic mastectomy was mentioned, Connie had become calmer and had immediately accepted it as the preferred course.

The surgeon felt that Connie's breasts were fairly easy to examine. She agreed that Connie's breast cancer risk did not appear to be great. When I reported my conversation with the surgeon to Connie, she said that *she* certainly had not wanted prophylactic mastectomy initially. She continued, "When the doctor suggested it the way she did, I thought it was serious or she would never even bring it up. When I heard her talk about prophylactic mastectomy, I knew I was in a dangerous situation and I just shut down." Connie's shutting down may have given the surgeon the impression that she was relieved and wanted surgery. Connie and her surgeon later had a long talk, realized that both were comfortable with careful surveillance, and did not schedule surgery. This is a clear example of the spiral of concern that I discussed in chapter 8. When emotional topics are discussed, anxiety can be generated in both doctor and patient, leading to an escalation of concern all around.

I've seen some women who initially state in strong terms that that they do not wish to have prophylactic mastectomy, but eventually do have the surgery and remain pleased with it. Usually these women become convinced that early detection will not work for them. This was the case with Suzanne, a woman in her early thirties, who was concerned about her breast cancer risk due to hereditary factors. Suzanne's breasts were quite dense on the mammogram, as is often the case in women her age. In addition, her breasts were large and, as she said, "filled with all kinds of lumps, cysts, and thickenings." She wanted to have children and feared that during pregnancy a breast cancer might grow to a large size before being detected. After much discussion and thought, she had both breasts removed. I have seen her several times in the years since. She is still comfortable with her choice and continues to feel she made the right decision:

> Having my breasts removed has eased my fears and helped me to feel that I'll live to raise my children. It was a very hard decision and I miss my breasts. But it was what I had to do.

Charlene also decided to have prophylactic mastectomies. Several of her father's sisters and her father's mother had been diagnosed with breast cancer at a young age. Her favorite aunt had died of the disease. At our first visit she said, "No body part is important enough to me to take the risk of dying the way my aunt did." We obtained the records on Charlene's aunt, which showed that her breast cancer was over 2 cm in size when it was found. Charlene recognized that with careful follow-up a breast cancer would probably be found in her breasts before it reached that size. Nevertheless, she continued to feel that prophylactic mastectomy was the right decision for her. After thinking about her options for some months she had her breasts removed and was pleased with her choice.

Prophylactic Mastectomy Guidelines

Over the years, I have developed increasing respect for a process in which information is provided in a careful, thoughtful manner and women are helped to use it. This process helps to ensure that women make the decisions that are right for them. Because it involves understanding new information and integrating it with old ideas and various emotional reactions that arise, it may take time and may require multiple visits to different specialists. If you are considering prophylactic mastectomy I hope you will continue your search until you are satisfied that you have learned enough to enable you to make the decisions that are right for you—not for your doctors or even for your family.

If you are considering prophylactic mastectomy, you are more likely to continue to feel comfortable with your choice over the years if all of the following apply:

- You find that your absolute breast cancer risk remains unacceptably high *to you,* even some months after you learn about it (and check to see how it was calculated).
- Several health care providers who specialize in breast disease tell you they believe that detection of a small breast cancer by mammography *and* physical breast examination would be very difficult or unlikely in your breasts.
- You understand the difference between the risk of being diagnosed with breast cancer and the chance of dying of it—in absolute terms. (Please refer to chapter 2 for a discussion of absolute risk.)
- You understand *that even with this surgery not all breast tissue can be removed.* Because not all breast tissue can be removed, cancer can still occur in tissue that remains after surgery. You will continue to need follow-up examinations and will need to check your breast and underarm areas for breast lumps.
- You discuss these issues with several health professionals who specialize in breast disease, your family, and friends, over several months. By allowing time for decision making, you have an opportunity to "try on" different approaches and change your mind several times before arriving at the decision that is right for you. This time is crucial.

If you use these criteria and then decide to go ahead with prophylactic mastectomy, you are likely to be far more comfortable with your choice, even years from now, than if you act more promptly "to get it over with so I can get on with my life."

The Drugs Tamoxifen and Raloxifene for Prevention

Tamoxifen

Tamoxifen is a drug that has long been used to treat women with breast cancer. More recently it has been studied in women *without* a breast cancer diagnosis to see if it could reduce their chances of developing a breast cancer. In the first large study of tamoxifen use by women who had not been diagnosed with breast cancer, those who took it had a 49% reduction in their chance of developing invasive breast cancer.[8] Many assumed that a 49% reduction in risk meant that the absolute or actual reduction in risk was also large. However, as you will see, the absolute risk is far smaller than the "49% reduction" might suggest on an intuitive level.

In this study, one group of about 6,500 women took tamoxifen for up to six years and about 6,500 women in another group did not take it. At the end of the 5.75 years of the study, 89 invasive breast cancers were found in the women who were taking tamoxifen. In the group who were not taking tamoxifen, 175 breast cancers were found.

Here it is important to note the 6,500 women in each group in order to keep in perspective the few numbers of breast cancers that were diagnosed in 5.75 years. And all of the women in this study were judged by the Gail model to have an increased breast cancer risk. In table 10.1, I summarize some of the study findings to help you put its results in perspective. You can see that the women who did not take tamoxifen had an annual average breast cancer rate of 0.6 *per 100 women,* compared to 0.3 per 100 women who took tamoxifen. That's a difference of only 0.3 *breast cancers per hundred women a year,* each year of the study. That is, on average fewer than one woman out of a hundred was diagnosed with breast cancer each year of the study—whether she took tamoxifen or not. And these women were all judged to be at high risk!

The results of the study can be presented in another way by considering risk from the beginning of the study up to 5.75 years—the time at which the study ended. Think of 100 women, each in her own car, driving along a highway. If all of these 100 women use a new type of brake (tamoxifen) every day for 5.75 years they can reduce the risk of accident (breast cancer) in their group from 3.8 to 2.0, as shown in the last row of table 10.1. If you subtract 2.0 from 3.8, you will see that at the end of 5.75 years the

TABLE 10.1

Breast Cancers in 5.75 Years
in Women Taking Tamoxifen for "Prevention"

Category	No Tamoxifen	Tamoxifen
Number of Women	6,599	6,575
Number of Breast Cancers	175	89
Average Annual Rate Per 100 Women	0.6	0.3
Rate Per 100 Women to 5.75 Years*	3.8	2.0

Source: Based on data from Fisher et al., 1998.

*The 1.8 difference per 100 women between the two groups means that 333 women would need to be treated for one year to avoid one breast cancer case.

entire group of 100 women with the new brake avoids 1.8 accidents (breast cancers). This means that if 100 high-risk women take tamoxifen, at the end of 5.75 years they will have 1.8 fewer breast cancers than another group that did not take tamoxifen. That's a reduction of 0.3 accident (breast cancer case) each year per 100 women. This example is based on the same data that produced the highly touted 49% reduction in risk.

Let's look at this one more way: How many women would need to take tamoxifen for one year to avoid one case of breast cancer in that year? Based on the number of breast cancers found in the two groups in this study, the answer is 333. Yes, 333 women would need to be treated with tamoxifen for one year to avoid one case of breast cancer in that year. That's what the 49% reduction found in this study means in absolute terms.

You may have noticed that I've been using the term *avoid* instead of *prevent* breast cancer in discussing this study's results. I do so because none of the women was studied long enough for scientists to be able to determine whether prevention actually occurred. Most breast cancers grow for seven to ten years before they are detected—longer than the 5.75 years of the study. Therefore, all, or almost all of the women who were diagnosed with breast cancer already had cancer before the start of the study and before any of them started taking tamoxifen. The study results, therefore, suggest that tamoxifen *might* delay, not prevent, the development of some breast cancers. The results do *not* provide evidence that tamoxifen "prevents" breast cancer.

Interestingly, tamoxifen studies in Europe have not obtained similar results. In the European studies, women who took tamoxifen did not have a reduction in breast cancer risk, even in comparison terms. Some speculate that differences between American and European women, smaller numbers of women in the European studies, or differences in methodology may have made it difficult to detect the small differences in risk that were present in the U.S. study. More studies will be needed to resolve these issues. For now, the main point is that *very small absolute differences in risk were found in the U.S. study between women who did and did not take tamoxifen*—1.8 per 100 women at the end of 5.75 years.

In addition to learning about the very small reduction in absolute risk for women without a breast cancer diagnosis who take tamoxifen, women who contemplate taking this drug need to be aware that its long-range effects, particularly on young women, are unknown. If a woman who takes tamoxifen should later develop breast cancer, we do not know whether tamoxifen will be useful in treating her cancer at that time. There are also short-term consequences, including menopausal symptoms such as sleeplessness, irritability, hot flashes, and aching joints. Women who take tamoxifen have a small increase in their risk of stroke, uterine cancer, blood clots in the lungs and veins, cataracts, and vaginal discharge. Many women report that their thought processes are less clear and that the world seems "fuzzy" while they are on tamoxifen.

In making a decision about whether to take tamoxifen you may find it useful to consider the following:

- The absolute difference in invasive breast cancer risk between women who did and did not take tamoxifen was 1.8 per 100 women at the end of 5.75 years.
- Studies in Europe do not find a decrease in breast cancer risk to women who take tamoxifen compared to those who do not take it.
- Some women who take tamoxifen experience side effects, including an increased risk of uterine cancer.

- The long-term effects of tamoxifen on healthy women are unknown.
- Tamoxifen has not been shown to *prevent* breast cancer.
- No study has found that tamoxifen reduces a woman's risk of death due to breast cancer.

Raloxifene

Raloxifene is a drug that is sometimes recommended to postmeno-pausal women to reduce their risk of osteoporosis* if they don't wish to take HRT. Women increasingly tell me that their doctors have suggested raloxifene as a way to reduce their breast cancer risk. Let's take a look at the data.

In one of the largest and longest studies, which lasted only 40 months, women who took raloxifene had a 76% reduction in breast cancer risk.[9] Again, many women (and physicians) assumed this meant that women who took raloxifene would have a sizable reduction in breast cancer risk. As with tamoxifen, the absolute reduction in breast cancer risk is quite small—2.7 cases per 1,000 woman years.† The authors of this study point out that 126 women would need to be treated with raloxifene for one year to avoid one case of breast cancer—in that year. This three-year study of raloxifene is one of the longest, so the long-term effect of this drug on healthy women is unknown.

When you consider the suspicion and skepticism with which the long-term studies of hormone replacement therapy are sometimes met, the ready acceptance of tamoxifen and raloxifene use with short-term studies is quite surprising. Scientists have studied hormone replacement therapy for over twenty years in groups of women with many different breast cancer risk factors. In contrast, we have information about the effects of tamoxifen and raloxifene on healthy women for less than six years. And women with various breast cancer risk factors who take these drugs have not been studied.

---

*Osteoporosis, the loss of bone that most frequently occurs in postmenopausal women, can result in a bent spine and an increased risk of bone fractures.
†"Woman-years" refers to the total number of years a group of women in a study has been followed. For example, ten women followed for one year equals ten years, as does one woman who is followed for ten years.

Guidelines for making decisions about tamoxifen and raloxifene are similar to those for prophylactic mastectomy, and include being aware of:

- Your own breast cancer risks, keeping in mind:
  - Flaws in the Gail model as well as its inappropriate use as an assessment of breast cancer risk to women who have a family history of breast cancer (discussed in chapter 9)
  - Your chance of finding breast cancer at a small size, when chemotherapy is generally not needed and the prognosis is usually excellent
- Known side effects of tamoxifen and raloxifene use
- Unknown long-term consequences of tamoxifen and raloxifene use
- The very, very small differences in absolute numbers of breast cancer that are found in women who do and do not take tamoxifen and raloxifene
- The failure of any study to show that the death rate due to breast cancer is decreased in women without a breast cancer diagnosis who take tamoxifen or raloxifene

Ovarian Cancer

Early Detection Methods

As you have seen, women with a family history of breast cancer sometimes have an increased risk of both breast and ovarian cancer. Ovarian cancer risks of up to 63% to age 70 for women with a BRCA1 mutation and 16% for those with a BRCA2 mutation have been reported. Women who have one of the three BRCA mutations most commonly found among individuals of Ashkenazi Jewish descent have been reported to have a 16% risk of ovarian cancer to age 70.

Unlike breast cancer, ovarian cancer is difficult to detect before it has spread. A 1994 National Institutes of Health panel of gynecologists concluded that the two methods most frequently used for early detection, transvaginal ultrasound and CA-125, did not reduce ovarian cancer mortality. In the most recent national figures, about 75% of ovarian cancers had spread by the time they were found.[10] The expected five-year survival for all ovarian cancers is currently about 44%. Because most ovarian cancers are not found at an early, curable stage, many women who are at increased risk consider having their ovaries removed as a way of reducing their chances of dying of this disease.

Prophylactic Oophorectomy

The removal of a woman's ovaries before she has been diagnosed with ovarian cancer (prophylactic oophorectomy) can be done laparoscopically.* Recovery time is far shorter than with a traditional hysterectomy.

Some have worried that women who have their ovaries removed might still be at increased risk of cancer of the peritoneum (the inner lining of the abdominal cavity), since the ovaries and the peritoneum are derived from the same embryologic tissue. More studies are needed to provide information about the risk of peritoneal cancer to women who have an increased risk of hereditary ovarian cancer. However, one of the largest studies of women who chose prophylactic oophorectomy is reassuring in this regard. In this study, over 300 women who had an increased risk of ovarian cancer due to strong hereditary factors had their ovaries removed prophylactically.[11] In the average sixteen years that these women were followed after their surgery, only 6 developed peritoneal cancer. Four of the six peritoneal cancers were found within five years of the time the women had their ovaries removed. Ovarian cancers are thought to grow for more than five years before they can be detected, so cancer was probably present in these four women at the time of their surgery. That leaves two peritoneal cancers that appear to have developed in over 300 women after their prophylactic oophorectomy.

Based on family history, the approximate number of ovarian cancers that would be expected to occur in this group is between 26 and 102, depending on the assumptions you make about the risk of ovarian cancer. In my calculations I assumed a lower risk of 16% and an upper risk of 63%, in keeping with current BRCA study results.

324 women × 50% (risk of carrying a mutation that increases cancer risk) = 162, the number likely to carry a mutation

---

*Laparoscopic surgery requires small incisions with small instruments. General anesthesia is used, but most women go home the same day.

162 × 16% (lower-risk estimate for developing ovarian cancer if a BRCA mutation is present) = 25.92

162 × 63% (upper estimate for developing ovarian cancer if a BRCA1 mutation is present) = 102

These calculations provide a rough approximation of the numbers of ovarian cancers that would be expected. Since only six (or two, if you count those that were unlikely to have been present at the time of surgery) women developed peritoneal cancer, this study suggests that surgery can reduce a woman's chances of developing ovarian cancer. More studies will be needed in this area before the risk of peritoneal cancer after oophorectomy is definitively known.

When women at increased risk of ovarian cancer have prophylactic surgery, it is recommended that their ovaries be checked thoroughly by a pathologist to be sure that no cancer cells are present in them. If you are contemplating prophylactic removal of your ovaries, you will probably find it useful to consult a gynecological oncologist to be sure that your surgery is conducted in a manner that is appropriate for a woman whose ovarian cancer risk is or might be increased. Before the surgery, you are also likely to benefit from a consultation with a gynecologist or endocrinologist who specializes in hormone replacement therapy to discuss the various options that are available to you, and to explore whether HRT is for you. This is particularly important if you are premenopausal when your ovaries are removed. Remember, the more information you have, the more perspectives you gain, the more capable you will be in making a decision that is right for you.

I also strongly recommend that you follow a process similar to that recommended for women who are contemplating prophylactic mastectomy. These guidelines are listed on page 203.

No matter how much risk and other information is available to us, no matter how carefully we live, uncertainty remains in all of our lives. For many of us, accepting and living with uncertainty can be a challenge. The women I see who face this challenge and pay attention to it generally find that they achieve a sense of peace and comfort, regardless of their risk, their family history, or their past experiences with cancer. In the next chapter I will discuss some of the ways my patients have achieved a greater sense of peace and security in the face of uncertainty.

Key Points to Remember

- The American Cancer Society recommends yearly mammograms for women from age 40 on.
- Since mammography does not find all breast cancers, physical breast examinations by a health professional every four to six months help many women live more comfortably with an increased breast cancer risk.
- Most breast cancers are found by women themselves, so breast self-examinations are an important part of a woman's follow-up program.
- Elements to consider in formulating your own breast care program include:
  - Information about your breast cancer risk
  - Information about prognosis if a breast cancer should be found
  - Help in moving through emotions that can act as barriers to understanding
  - Information about early detection methods and so-called means of prevention.
- If you are considering prophylactic mastectomy, be sure to
  - Learn your risks
  - Ask several health professionals about the chance of finding a cancer in your breast before it has spread
  - Remember that cancer can occur in the breast area after surgery, so you will continue to need checkups
  - Allow time in which to consider the new information and work through any emotional reactions to it.
- If you are considering taking tamoxifen to reduce breast cancer risk, remember that:
  - The actual number of breast cancers was reduced by 1.8 *per 100* women in the only study that has found a difference in risk between women who do and do not take tamoxifen
  - Based on the results of this study, 333 women would need to be

treated with tamoxifen for one year to avoid one case of breast cancer

- The long-term effects of tamoxifen use are unknown
- The future effectiveness of tamoxifen if breast cancer should be diagnosed is unknown
- Tamoxifen use has not been found to reduce breast cancer mortality.
- If you are considering taking raloxifene to reduce risk, remember that:
  - Long-term effects are unknown
  - Breast cancer risk is reduced by only 2.7 cases *per 1,000 woman years*
  - 126 women would need to be treated for one year to avoid one case of breast cancer.
- If you have concerns about ovarian cancer risk, use the elements suggested for prophylactic mastectomy in considering prophylactic oophorectomy, and also remember that:
  - Most ovarian cancers have spread by the time they are found
  - In the largest study to date of women who had prophylactic oophorectomy, very few later developed peritoneal cancer.

ELEVEN

Living at Ease with Uncertainty

The mind is its own place, and in itself
Can make a Heav'n of Hell, a Hell of Heav'n
What matter where, if I be still the same.

John Milton, *Paradise Lost*

These words are spoken ironically by the Devil in Milton's *Paradise Lost*. Yet they remind me of the very real state of some of my patients. Even years after their relative, a friend, or they themselves were diagnosed with breast cancer, they may still be suffering as a result of it. No matter how well or prosperous they are in many aspects of their life, they say that the uncertainty, the not knowing "when I'll get cancer" or feeling that they are "living with a sword over my head" greatly diminishes the quality of their lives.

We all live in an uncertain world. We realize, at least intellectually, that we could become ill or even die at any moment. Mostly, though, we banish uncertainty to some other less conscious part of our minds, or we do our best to avoid thoughts about future illness and our own mortality. Women who have experienced breast cancer, even in a friend or relative, sometimes have a more heightened awareness of life's uncertainty than others who have not had such an experience. For some, uncertainty can loom so large that it interferes with the enjoyment of life. This is particularly so when a woman feels that there is no way out—that she is "doomed to get breast cancer" or that she will inevitably follow the same course as her friend or relative who was diagnosed with it.

Some women are traumatized by their experiences with breast cancer, even though the term "trauma" is rarely used to describe what has happened to them. As a result, a news item, hearing about someone diagnosed with breast cancer, feeling what might be a new lump in her breast, can produce considerable and long-lasting anxiety. Many tell me they are angry with themselves for "letting these feelings take over," but also acknowledge that they feel powerless to stop them. This type of persistent and strong sense of danger is a normal outgrowth of trauma.

If you have been traumatized or deeply affected, you may know intellectually that the danger to you is not as high as you genuinely feel it to be, but you may find it difficult to put your fear or concern in perspective— at least sometimes. If you have been told or if you feel that you are at "high risk," how do you get on with your life while you are "waiting for the other shoe to drop"? How do you go beyond feeling "I know I'll never recover emotionally" or "I know I'll always be anxious about cancer"?

This chapter presents a summary of some of the ways my patients, who were or who felt they had a high breast cancer risk, have coped with their feelings about uncertainty. No one way works for all, so here I describe several different approaches for you to explore. To evaluate the effectiveness of a method, you will probably need to use it for at least six months. And, of course, the exercises described will work only if you set time aside to do them. Reading about them, thinking about them, and talking about them are no substitute for action.

You may well find, as many of my patients have, that the following three steps help you to start:

1. Reminding yourself about new information pertaining to a woman's excellent prognosis when a breast cancer is found at a small size

2. Setting up a breast health program with appropriate health care professionals that feels reasonable and effective

3. Training your mind

I discuss each of the above topics in this chapter. I offer these approaches to you with great confidence in their ability to help, since I have seen the increase in peace and enjoyment of life that they have brought to those of my patients who used them.

Step I: Remembering the Information

❧ When you feel yourself becoming uneasy about your breast cancer risk and its consequences to you, it's important to remind yourself of the difference between your situation and that of women who were diagnosed with breast cancer in the past. Even a quick reminder of some of the differences and new information about prognosis is likely to help, particularly if you make a list of the points most relevant to you. Keep the list handy so you can read and remember it when you first have a sense of unease.

Each person's list is likely to be somewhat different, of course. Here are examples of some of the types of information you might want to have on your reminder list:

- A woman's chances of dying of breast cancer have been decreasing since 1989.
- For breast cancers up to 1 cm in size that have not spread to the lymph nodes under the arm (and most have not), the survival all the way up to twenty years is 92%.
- Mammography and thorough physical breast examinations can often find breast cancers that are less than 1 cm in size.
- Improved techniques to detect small breast cancers are being developed.
- Now that you have learned how to evaluate risk, you are better prepared to evaluate the significance of new information as it becomes available. You can therefore feel more confident in your ability to appreciate the significance of important information. And you are less likely to be misled.
- You now know about the workings of the health care system as it pertains to the early detection and treatment of breast cancer, including the types of doctors to see and the services to obtain to best protect your health.
- Even if you are someone whose mother's breast cancer was due to strong hereditary factors, you are not destined to follow the same course, since you are not her genetic clone. You have half your mother's genes, not all of them. Also, you have opportunities for early

detection and for improved treatments that were not available even a few years ago.

You will probably find it helpful to take time over the next few days— and after—to produce your own list, and add to it when you think of new, useful items. Keep it close so you can read through it at a moment's notice. The sooner you remind yourself of these points the better.

Step II: Setting Up a Health Plan

To best safeguard your health and your peace of mind, it's important to take time to evaluate your breast health care program to be sure it meets your current needs. If it does not, you may want to set aside some time each week to explore other options. Talk to friends, relatives, and coworkers about their breast health care providers. You might call organizations such as the American Cancer Society or your local breast center to learn about available services and programs.

Once you have located prospective health professionals and services, take time to visit them to evaluate the care each is able to provide. At this point, remember that you are interviewing potential new employees to see which will suit you. Be sure to ask about cost. Some of my patients have been surprised to learn that they could afford to pay for breast examinations from health professionals who were not on their health plan. The money they spent was well worth it to these women, since they felt they were receiving the type of care they wanted and that would best help to protect their health.

In this endeavor it's important to persevere and avoid being discouraged if you don't immediately find the health practitioners or services you would like. Even if you have to search for three or six months to find the health care professionals and services that are right for you, the time will have been well spent. And remember also that if you set aside only 30 minutes each week to investigate your options, you will accomplish a great deal in several months. You don't have to do it all at once.

Step III: Mind Training

In our society, it's interesting how little we think about or talk seriously about training our minds. I often see women who think nothing of spending hours a week in the gym, running, or training for a tennis tournament or swim meet. Some go regularly to fitness classes. Some tell me why, due to past *physical* traumas, they are focusing on strengthening particular muscles. They fully and quite reasonably expect that with time and with disciplined, concerted effort they will change the way their bodies respond. Yet when it comes to our minds we tend to accept that we are stuck with our current emotions, sensitivities, or outlook. We recognize that past experiences have helped to shape the way we are at present and may even point to past events or to the influence of certain people in shaping how we feel and react. Even so, we often forget that just as with our bodies, it is possible to strengthen and reshape our minds, no matter how difficult our past has been.

My patients' experiences provide excellent examples of the extent to which a person's thoughts, anxieties, concerns, fear, and even feelings of doom can change. Following are four approaches my patients have used to train their minds so that their fears, worries, concerns, misgivings, and even feelings of helplessness or hopelessness became less prominent in their lives. You are welcome to try them and to adapt them to your life and situation. Remember, as with the development of any skill, you will need to practice to obtain results. And like muscle training, it's wise to start with a doable, realistic level and build steadily from there.

Approach 1: Noticing

Sometimes our fears or concerns are so unpleasant that we push them aside, hoping they will disappear. In time, the habit of pushing aside can become so automatic we may not be consciously aware of the uncomfortable thought or feeling residing inside us or may not be aware of the extent to which it is influencing our lives. The first inkling we have that all is not well may be an unexpected outburst, a feeling of irritability that "arises from nowhere," a tense back or shoulder, an upset stomach, or a headache.

The first step, then, is to notice your thoughts, feelings, and reactions over time. You might carry a small notebook with you to *very briefly* record what you are thinking and feeling, and to notice what your physical sensations are at a particular time. If you have access to a timer or some other way to be reminded to check in at unexpected times, you may learn a great deal about thoughts, feelings, and physical sensations that you hadn't realized were present or hadn't realized were present to the extent they are. Just set the timer and forget about it until it reminds you to notice the state of your body and mind. Many people find that their habitual thoughts and emotions have become so familiar that they are no longer consciously aware of them.

When you have kept these brief notes for several weeks, you might sit down and look for patterns. (Since you are looking for patterns, it's less useful to scrutinize the results every day.) You might find, for example, that stories about breast cancer in the newspaper produce a slight unease in your stomach or that when you are experiencing difficulty at work, your throat tightens and you become a bit worried about breast cancer risk. Even if your thoughts or physical sensations are fleeting or don't seem to have meaning, continue! The point of this exercise is to keep noticing. Over time you will see patterns in your reactions and will have a better understanding of the way in which you react.

Once you are better informed about the details, you are likely to find that ideas about how to ease your situation will occur to you. Or, as many have told me, the more they "saw" of what they were thinking and feeling the more these troublesome aspects melted away. Often it is just those times of the day or week when you are too busy or too involved to do this exercise that some of the more interesting material may appear. So, as much as possible, stick to the schedule that you have set for yourself. Even if you do this exercise only one day a week or most of one day a week, you are likely to reap great benefits.

I've put this exercise first because of its fundamental importance. Until you notice what is going on, until you become aware of the *details* of your uncomfortable thoughts and feelings, you may be hampered in effectively lessening them. Some feelings are so painful that most of us glance at them from the corners of our eyes and avoid examining them closely. They are simply too unpleasant for us to dwell on them. As Daniel Goleman notes in *Vital Lies, Simple Truths:* "The brain . . . has the ability to bear pain by masking its sting, but at the cost of a diminished awareness."[1] He continues, "To put it in the form of one of R. D. Laing's *Knots:*"

The range of what we think and do
is limited by what we fail to notice.
And because we fail to notice
that we fail to notice
there is little we can do
to change
until we notice
how failing to notice
shapes our thoughts and deeds

The noticing exercise is designed to help you begin to see the details of what you may have failed to see or failed to see clearly.

Approach 2: Replacing

One way to help reduce anxious or fearful thoughts that you have determined are baggage from the past and *that do not require current thought or action* is to replace them with pleasant, peaceful thoughts. With practice, you will be amazed to find that your thoughts will increasingly tend to go along the new, more positive track instead of the old, with its feelings of doom and gloom. This occurs because in some ways the mind is quite simple. As a worry continues, it's as if it etches a channel into the ground. With continued worry the channel gets deeper and deeper, making it easier for your thoughts to fall into an ever deepening "doom" trench and more difficult for them to escape.

When you begin to replace the old habitual thoughts and anxieties with pleasant, hopeful thoughts, you are helping to establish new channels. In time, your thoughts will quite naturally tend to follow the new channels instead of the old. For example, when feelings of concern about breast cancer risk come up, you can replace them with a reminder that early breast cancer detection is now more possible and then turn your thoughts to other more hopeful and pleasant topics in your life that are not related to uncertainty or to breast cancer.

I am *not* suggesting that you replace every concern, every anxiety in your life with a pleasant thought. I am *not* encouraging you to deny or to cover up all of your thoughts and feelings. Instead, when you have rationally decided that you have done all that you can about a concern, such as a concern about breast cancer risk, and the concern still remains, the replacement exercise is often useful. At other times your feelings of concern may be one way you have of knowing that further decisions and perhaps further actions are warranted.

Some women attempt to cope with difficult thoughts and feelings by denying them or pushing them away. One way to do this is to stay very busy, as Samantha did: "I do a lot of things and I'm not sure it's real healthy for me. I think I'm double-timing or triple-timing even. It's another way of being an ostrich."

These women often pay a high price for their denial, as Joanna Macy points out in her book, *World as Lover, World as Self:*

> The refusal to feel takes a heavy toll. Not only is there an impoverishment of our emotional and sensory life—flowers are dimmer and less fragrant, our loves less ecstatic—but this psychic numbing also impedes our capacity to process and respond to information.[2]

As you do the replacement exercise, you may initially find that your thoughts or emotions are so upsetting that it is sometimes uncomfortable to proceed. However, if you persist, even for short periods, every day for three months, you are likely to find that the exercise does work and that you have not been overwhelmed by anxious thoughts. Remember not to take on more than you can do at any one time. If you do, you may find that you have the equivalent of sore abdominal muscles after doing too many sit-ups. And, in a day or so, like the sore abdominal muscles, the "overdone" emotions will calm also.

Actually, the replacement exercise can help you to become better acquainted with painful thoughts and feelings without being consumed or overwhelmed by them. For example, if you have an injured leg and are feeling a great desire to run, you probably won't do so if it will result in further damage. In this case you don't deny that you have a strong feeling about wanting to exercise, but you also don't act on it or allow the feeling to take you over, either. Instead, you remind yourself of the larger picture—the speedy recovery of your leg—and turn your thoughts elsewhere to more pleasant topics. I'm suggesting the same type of approach when you experience a painful emotion associated with uncertainty and breast cancer risk.

You may wonder how it is possible to experience emotions such as fear or concern without being taken over by them. With practice, people find that they can remind themselves of the larger picture in a way that is similar to that described in the leg injury example. They find they can stand back or stand to one side of their difficult feelings, as if they were watching the action from the sidelines instead of being in the middle of the field. In time, the troublesome emotions are likely to take up a smaller and smaller space as they are replaced with more and more frequent pleasant thoughts. As this happens, the part of you that is watching has more and more room in which to be comfortable, because there are more pleasant feelings. Again, the point is not to cover up or deny the unpleasant sensations, but to recognize them when they come up, see them for what they are (in this example, not a call for current action, but hangers-on from the past), and realize that they are *part* of what is happening and are not the whole of your life, even at that moment. My patients who stick with this exercise often reap enormous benefits, particularly if they realize that what they are thinking and feeling is an outgrowth of their past experiences and is not due to any inherent fault in them.

Inventiveness seems to help also. For example, some found that they are greatly helped by keeping a daily account of what is going well in their life, large and small: the people who help, those who give them a smile, an interesting bird or flower, or a walk with a friend. Then, when difficult or unpleasant feelings arise, they are able to go back to this account to remind themselves of all that is going well—items that are all too easy to forget in the midst of our busy lives. Because unpleasant or uneasy feelings often have their origin in and were shaped by past experiences, they can be reshaped by new thoughts and experiences. It's fine in this regard to act as your own trainer or coach and create new exercises and new incentives for yourself as needed.

Some find that when they experience any unpleasant emotion it helps to stay with that feeling for even a breath or two, breathing in the unpleasant feeling to the full extent possible, then breathing out a sense of release, peace, and contentment—breathing in and breathing out. In this way, they find that difficult feelings subside more rapidly. This approach may seem paradoxical, but it can definitely help to diminish painful feelings and increase a person's sense of well-being.[3] The major difficulty with this exercise may be in reminding yourself to do it when you are feeling unsettled. So you might want to choose several times a day to practice on whatever you are feeling at that moment. Once you are accustomed to doing this exercise, you are more likely to remember it when your feelings are particularly strong.

To bring about healing from painful thoughts and feelings that have their origin in the past, it is often useful to focus on currently held beliefs that have arisen from them. One very effective approach, called the Option Dialogue Process, makes use of a series of nonjudgmental questions to help individuals better understand their beliefs, since "Each person does the best they can in accordance with their beliefs. Change the beliefs and the resulting feelings and behaviors change."[4]

Until a person is clear about what her beliefs actually are, however, they can literally run her life from behind the scenes. For example, in this book you have seen how valuable information can be in correcting misinformation, which in turn can lead to misbeliefs. Similarly, by helping in the exploration of these and other beliefs, the Option process can be enormously liberating.

Approach 3: Deep Relaxation

Deep relaxation and meditation both help to quiet the conscious mind. When this occurs, your thoughts and feelings may be more clearly understood and appreciated. These processes can help you to untangle old, persistent ways of thinking, believing, and behaving.

Guided meditation tapes for relaxation and for directed topics such as anxiety reduction are widely available. Some are, of course, far more effective than others. See what works for you. But remember, you will need to practice and repeat. And you may need to search a bit to find an approach that suits you. The value of good "navigational practices" and second opinions discussed in chapter 8 holds in this area also.

Some of my patients have made their own deep relaxation tapes. Before relaxing they make a tape with a message they would like their system to "get," such as feeling more peaceful and relaxed. The most effective messages seem to be those that are put in positive terms. So instead of saying, "I want less fear," you might say something like, "I want to realize that I have taken all the right steps to protect myself, and that I am now in a safe place. I want to feel the peace appropriate to that place."

To become more relaxed, sit in a quiet, comfortable place with your back straight and your feet on the floor. You may feel more at ease if you ask part of yourself to remain alert so it can take care of any problem that should require your attention while you are relaxing. Ask that part to rouse you immediately if your attention should be needed. Then breathe in an easy manner. There are several ways to proceed from here. I'll describe one that seems to have been useful to many people. Put your left thumb and first finger together gently. (This is a way to help your body remember to relax in the future.) In your right hand, hold a pencil or pen loosely between your fingers. Then, starting with your feet, relax on an exhale. As you continue breathing, with each exhale relax your feet, legs, and so on up through your body in sections, ending with your head. With each exhale tell yourself to relax and focus on relaxing that part of your body. If a body part is particularly tense, you may want to stay with it for several breaths. At first, focus on small sections of your body. Later you will need fewer breaths to relax your whole body.

Once you have relaxed your body, think of a comfortable and enjoyable place and imagine yourself there. Feel all the details of the place: the air on your skin, the sights, the smells, and the sounds. Imagine that you are joined by someone dear to you. As you continue to imagine yourself in the pleasant place you have chosen, you will relax more and more. At some point you will find that the pencil drops from between your fingers. When it does, place your hand flat on your lap. Especially at first, you may need some time and practice in relaxing before the pencil drops. Persist!

If you follow this approach two or three times a day for several days, you will find that with practice you will relax enough for the pencil to drop. When it does, tell yourself "deeper, deeper" to relax even more deeply. Once you are in a deeply relaxed state, you many want to simply rest there and enjoy the peace. Some women tell me that the messages they give themselves, such as permission to relax, to feel at peace, to realize that they are taking care of their breast health care in the most effective manner possible, really sink in when they are in a fully relaxed state, and that the effect of these messages lasts for some time. And, of course, over time the messages you give yourself may change. Here again it is important to be creative. Or you may want to play a relaxation tape—your own, or one you have found useful.

Approach 4: Meditation

Many people find that meditation greatly helps to reduce stress and calms their minds so they can "hear and feel" their rapidly changing thoughts, feelings, and bodily states. From this approach comes a heightened sense of peace and well-being. There are many different types of meditation and countless books describing them. Here I'll merely talk about a basic approach to this important area. To begin, find a quiet, comfortable place to sit, with your back straight and your feet flat on the floor. Then, pay attention to your breath as it leaves your nose. As you do, thoughts and feelings will quite naturally come to your attention. When your mind wanders, return to your breath as a way of staying focused on your body and calming and training your mind.

You may also find it useful to *briefly* label the type of thought you have before you return to your breath—for example, planning, fearing, wishing, wondering, and so forth. In time, usually with the help of a more experienced meditator, those who regularly practice this approach achieve an increased sense of peace and security. There are many books describing a number of approaches to meditation, since no one approach suits all. As with the replacement exercise, meditation works most effectively if you do it regularly for some months. Start with just a few minutes once or twice a day at scheduled times and build up. You'll be surprised how pleasurable and helpful this approach can be.

Moving Forward

When women recount the times that have given rise to their fiercest thoughts, feelings, and fears, they often say that these times have been their most valuable teachers. When I ask what they learned, they say that they are now more likely to live in the present, to enjoy their life, and to be aware of their priorities. They are less likely to become upset when life doesn't go the way they would like or expect. Some say that as a result of their experiences they have a deeper empathy for others and for whatever problems or troubles another person may be having. Suzanne put it this way:

> I don't mean to sound corny. But now I know that I can weather just about anything that comes along in life. And I can find some way to have joy in my life every day no matter what. And I used to be so frightened all the time!

I hope that the information in this book will help you, as it helped Suzanne, to find joy in life each day "no matter what." This may be more likely to occur if you remember, as discussed earlier in this book, to:

- Distinguish between the risk of a breast cancer diagnosis and the chance of dying of it.
- Use the tools for assessing risk that you learned here to assess new study results.
- Keep in mind that women whose breast cancers are found at a small size have an excellent prognosis.
- Find health professionals to help you implement a breast health program that seems reasonable to you.
- Use mind training approaches such as those discussed here to help you live more comfortably with uncertainty.

Above all, please be kind to yourself. Your current thoughts and feelings had their origin in your past life experiences, so new experiences, including learning about the tools described in this book, can change them.

APPENDIX A

❧❧

Questionnaires to Determine
If You Might Benefit from
Cancer Risk Assessment

The questionnaires in this section are designed to help you determine if you would be likely to benefit from Cancer Risk Assessment. If you answer yes to any of the following questions you may find it useful to seek Cancer Risk Assessment from a geneticist or genetic counselor.

Since most cancers are *not* due to strong hereditary factors, a "yes" answer is not proof that your hereditary cancer risk is increased—only that you are likely to benefit from a risk analysis. Remember also that if you answer "no" to all the questions there is no guarantee that your risk of cancer due to hereditary factors is not increased.

FOR WOMEN WITH A
FAMILY HISTORY OF BREAST CANCER

	Yes	No
1. Were two relatives on one side of your family diagnosed with breast cancer, with one of them your mother or your aunt?	_____	_____
2. Were three or more of your relatives on one side of your family diagnosed with breast cancer?	_____	_____
3. Was one of your relatives diagnosed with ovarian cancer?	_____	_____
4. Have two of your relatives been diagnosed with breast cancer and one or more with another cancer?	_____	_____
5. Was one of your relatives diagnosed with more than one cancer?	_____	_____
6. Were two generations on either side of your family diagnosed with cancer?	_____	_____
7. Do you have a male relative who was diagnosed with breast cancer?	_____	_____
8. Do you have a relative who was diagnosed with cancer before age 50?	_____	_____

FOR WOMEN DIAGNOSED WITH BREAST CANCER

A. If None of Your Relatives Was Diagnosed with Cancer

	Yes	No
1. Were you diagnosed with breast cancer before age 50?	_____	_____
2. Have you had cancer in both breasts?	_____	_____
3. Have you had another (non-breast) cancer?	_____	_____

B. If One or More of Your Relatives Was Diagnosed with Cancer

	Yes	No
1. Were you or a relative diagnosed with cancer before age 50?	____	____
2. Were two or more of your relatives diagnosed with breast cancer?	____	____
3. Was one of your relatives diagnosed with ovarian cancer?	____	____
4. Have you had another (non-breast) cancer?	____	____
5. Did one of your relatives have breast cancer and another a different cancer?	____	____
6. Did your mother or father die (of any cause) before age 45?	____	____
7. Were two generations on either side of your family diagnosed with cancer?	____	____
8. Do you have a male relative who was diagnosed with breast cancer?	____	____

FOR WOMEN DIAGNOSED WITH OVARIAN CANCER

	Yes	No
1. Do you have a relative (parent, sibling, child, grandparent, uncle, aunt, niece, nephew, grandchild) who was diagnosed with		
• breast cancer?	____	____
• ovarian cancer (if a woman)?	____	____
2. Are you of Ashkenazi Jewish descent?	____	____
3. Have you been diagnosed with another type of cancer?	____	____
4. Are you less than 55 years old?	____	____

Where to Go for Breast and Ovarian Cancer Risk Information

Web Sites

- Cancer Risk Assessment and Counseling: www.dnai.com/~ptkelly
- PubMed: www.nc.bi.nlm.nih.gov/PubMed
- The Breast Cancer.Net Newsletter: www.breastcancer.net

Organizations

- National Society of Genetic Counselors: 610-872-7608; www.nsgc.org
- Cancer Information Service: 800-4-CANCER
- Oncology Nursing Society: 412-921-7373; www.ons.org
- North American Menopause Society: 440-442-7550; www.menopause.org

Glossary

Absolute risk: Risk over time; risk that is not based on a comparison with another group's risk.

Benign: Non-cancerous.

Benign breast disease: See fibrocystic breast disease.

Biopsy: Removal of tissue.

Chromosome: Long stringlike structures in the nucleus of a cell; genes are located on the chromosomes.

Cyst: Fluid-filled sac.

Cytoplasm: Part of the cell that does not contain the nucleus.

DNA: Deoxyribonucleic acid, chemicals that compose the genes.

Excision: Removal of tissue when all of a particular area or lump is removed.

Fibrocystic breast disease: Changes in breast tissue; most do not increase breast cancer risk; sometimes called benign breast disease.

Genes: Strings of chemicals that have the ability to make other chemicals that cause growth and development.

Genetic: Refers to genes in any cell; often confused with heredity. Only genetic changes that occur in the eggs or sperm can be inherited. These are called hereditary changes.

Hereditary: Genetic change that can be inherited.

Heterogeneous: A mixed group, as in women who have different types of fibrocystic breast disease.

Hormone: Chemical produced in one part of the body that travels through the blood to another body part where it produces an effect, e.g., estrogen.

Hyperplasia of breast: Minor changes to cells lining the terminal ductolobular unit.

Metastasis: Spread of cancer cells from cancerous tumor to another body part.

Mutation: Change in a gene's chemicals.

Nucleus: Part of the cell containing the chromosomes.

Oncology: Study of cancer.

Proliferative disease of the breast: See hyperplasia.

Somatic cell: A non-egg or non-sperm cell; mutations in somatic cells are not inherited.

Tamoxifen: A drug sometimes used to treat women with invasive breast cancer; more recently suggested for women at "increased" breast cancer risk.

Terminal ducto-lobular unit: Part of the breast duct structure in which breast cancer arises.

Notes

Chapter 1

1. Stuart-Brown S and Farmer A. Screening could seriously damage your health. *BMJ* 314:533–34, 1997.

Chapter 2

1. Cole KC. *The Universe and the Teacup: The Mathematics of Truth and Beauty.* New York, Harcourt Brace, 1997.

2. Ries LAG, Kosary CL, Hankey BF et al., eds. *SEER Cancer Statistics Review, 1973–1996.* National Cancer Institute, Bethesda, Md., 1999.

3. Tabar L, Duffy SW, Vitak B et al. The natural history of breast carcinoma. *Cancer* 86:449–62, 1999.

4. Lopez MJ and Smart CR. Twenty-year follow-up of minimal breast cancer from the breast cancer detection demonstration project. *Surg Onc Clin N Am* 6:393–401, 1997.

5. Arnesson LG, Smeds S, Fagerberg G. Recurrence-free survival in patients with small breast cancer. *Eur J Surg* 160:271–76, 1994.

6. Joensuu H, Pylkkanen L, Toikkanen S. Late mortality from T1N0M0 breast carcinoma. *Cancer* 85:2183–89, 1999.

7. Claus EB, Risch NJ, and Thompson WD. Age at onset as an indicator of familial risk of breast cancer. *Am J Epid* 131:961–72, 1990.

8. Anderson DE and Badzioch MD. Risk of familial breast cancer. *Cancer* 56:383–87, 1985.

Chapter 3

1. Sontag S. *Illness As Metaphor.* New York, Farrar, Straus & Giroux, 1988.

2. Sonnenschein C and Soto AM. *The Society of Cells.* New York, Springer-Verlag, 1999.

3. Ibid.

Chapter 4

1. Ford D, Easton DF, Bishop DT et al. Risks of cancer in BRCA1-mutation carriers. *Lancet* 343:692–95, 1994; Easton DF, Ford D, Bishop DT et al. Breast and ovarian cancer incidence in BRCA1-mutation carriers. *Am J Hum Genet* 56:265–71, 1995.

2. Breast Cancer Linkage Consortium. Cancer risks in BRCA2 mutation carriers. *J Natl Cancer Inst* 91:1310–16, 1999.

3. Easton DF, Ford D, Bishop DT et al. Ibid.

4. Ford D, Easton DF et al. Ibid.

5. Breast Cancer Linkage Consortium. Ibid.

6. Ries LAG, Kosary CL, Hankey BF et al., eds. *SEER Cancer Statistics Review, 1973–1996.* National Cancer Institute, Bethesda, Md., 1999.

7. NIH Consensus Development Panel. 1994.

8. Struewing JP, Hartge P, Wacholder S et al. The risk of cancer associated with specific mutations of BRCA1 and BRCA2 among Ashkenazi Jews. *New Engl J Med* 336:1401–8, 1997.

9. Begg CB, Satagopan JM, Robson M et al. Lifetime breast cancer risk associated with BRCA1 and BRCA2 mutations among patients of Ashkenazi Jewish origin. *Am J Hum Genet* 65:A61, 1999.

10. Struewing JP, Hartge P, Wacholder S et al. Ibid.

11. Collins, FS. BRCA1: Lots of mutations, lots of dilemmas. *NEJM* 334:186–88, 1996.

12. Tonin P, Weber B, Offit K et al. Frequency of recurrent BRCA1 and BRCA2 mutations in Ashkenazi Jewish breast cancer families. *Nature Medicine* 2:1179–83, 1996.

13. Breast Cancer Linkage Consortium. Ibid.

14. Anderson, DE and Badzioch MD. Bilaterality in familial breast cancer patients. *Cancer* 56:2092–98, 1985.

15. Frank TS, Manley SA, Olufunmilayo I et al. Sequence analysis of BRCA1 and BRCA2: Correlation of mutations with family history and ovarian cancer risk. *J Clin Oncol* 16:2417–25, 1998.

Chapter 5

1. Tomaszewski JE and LiVolsi VA. Mandatory second opinion of pathologic slides: Is it necessary? *Cancer* 86:2198–200, 1999.

2. Page DL, Dupont WD, Rogers LW et al. Atypical hyperplastic lesions of the

female breast. *Cancer* 55:2698–708, 1985; Dupont WD and Page DL. Risk factors for breast cancer in women with proliferative breast disease. *New Engl J Med* 312:146–51, 1985; Bodian CA, Perzin KH, Lattes R et al. Prognostic significance of benign proliferative breast disease. *Cancer* 71:3896–907, 1993.

3. Page DL et al. Ibid.

4. Bodian CA et al. Ibid.

5. Page DL et al. Ibid.

6. Fechner RE. History of ductal carcinoma in situ. In: *Ductal Carcinoma In Situ of the Breast,* Silverstein MJ, ed. Baltimore, Williams and Wilkins, 1997, pp. 13–21.

7. Ibid.

8. Lininger RA and Tavassoli FA. Atypical intraductal hyperplasia of the breast. In: *Ductal Carcinoma In Situ of the Breast,* Silverstein, MJ, ed. Baltimore, Williams and Wilkins, 1997, pp. 195–222.

9. Foucar E. Carcinoma-in-situ of the breast: Have pathologists run amok? *Lancet* 347:707–8, 1996.

10. Lininger RA and Tavassoli FA. Ibid.

11. Fechner RE. Ibid.

12. Silverstein MJ, Rosser RJ, Gierson ED et al. Axillary lymph mode dissection for intraductal breast carcinoma: Is it indicated? *Cancer* 59:1819–24, 1987.

13. Silverstein MJ. Ductal carcinoma in situ with microinvasion. In: *Ductal Carcinoma In Situ of the Breast,* Silverstein, MJ, ed. Baltimore, Williams and Wilkins, 1997b, pp. 557–62.

14. Welch HG and Black WC. Using autopsy series to estimate the disease "reservoir" for ductal carcinoma in situ of the breast: How much more breast cancer can we find? *Ann Intern Med* 127:1023–28, 1997.

15. Page DL and Dupont WD. Indicators of increased breast cancer risk in humans. *J Cell Biochem* 16GSuppl: 175–82, 1992.

16 Silverstein MJ, Lagios MD, Craig PH et al. A prognostic index for ductal carcinoma in situ of the breast. *Cancer* 77:2267–74, 1996; Lagios MD and Silverstein MJ. Ductal carcinoma in situ: The success of breast conservation therapy: a shared experience of two single institutional nonrandomized prospective studies. *Surg Oncol Clin N Am* 6:385–92, 1997.

17. Lagios MD, Margolin FR, Westdahl PR et al. Mammographically detected duct carcinoma in situ. *Cancer* 63:618–24, 1989.

18. Silverstein MJ. In: *Ductal Carcinoma In Situ of the Breast,* Silverstein MJ, ed. Baltimore, Williams and Wilkins, 1997a, pp. 271–83.

19. Silverstein MJ, Poller DN, Waisman JR et al. Prognostic classification of breast ductal carcinoma-in-situ. *Lancet* 345:1154–57, 1995.

20. Silverstein MJ, Lagios MD, Groshen S et al. The influence of margin width on local control of ductal carcinoma in situ of the breast. *New Engl J Med* 340:1455–61, 1999.

21. Lagios MD and Silverstein MJ. Ibid.

22. Silverstein MJ, Poller DN et al. Ibid.

23. Lagios MD, Westdahl PR, Margolin FR et al. Duct carcinoma in situ: Relationship of extent of noninvasive disease to the frequency of occult invasion, multicentricity, lymph node metastases, and short-term treatment failures. *Cancer* 50:1309–14, 1982.

24. Fisher B, Dignam J, Wolmark N et al. Lumpectomy and radiation therapy for the treatment of intraductal breast cancer: Findings from National Surgical Adjuvant Breast and Bowel Project B-17. *J Clin Oncol* 16: 441–52, 1998.

25. Schwartz GF. Treatment of subclinical and ductal carcinoma in situ by local excision and surveillance: A personal experience. In: *Ductal Carcinoma In Situ of the Breast.* Silverstein MJ, ed. Baltimore, Williams and Wilkins, 1997, pp. 353–60.

26. Page DL and Lagios MD. Pathologic analysis of the national surgical adjuvant breast Project (NSABP) B-17 trial. *Cancer* 75:1219–22, 1995.

27. Silverstein MJ, Lagios MD, Craig PH et al. Ibid.

28. Silverstein MJ and Lagios MD. Use of predictors of recurrence to plan therapy for DCIS of the breast. *Oncology* 11:393–410, 1997.

29. Lagios MD and Silverstein MJ. Ibid.

30. Silverstein MJ and Lagios MD, Groshen S et al. Ibid.

31. Fisher B, Dignam J, Wolmark N et al. Tamoxifen in treatment of intraductal breast cancer: National Surgical Adjuvant Breast and Bowel Project B-24 randomised controlled trial. *Lancet* 353:1993–2000, 1999.

32. Lagios MD. Classification of duct carcinoma in situ (DCIS) with a characterization of high-grade lesions. Defining cohorts for chemoprevention trials. *J Cell Biochem* 25S: 108–11, 1996.

33. Silverstein MJ, Lagios MD et al. Ibid.

34. Haagensen CD, Lane N, Lattes R et al. Lobular neoplasia (so-called lobular carcinoma in situ) of the breast. *Cancer* 42:737–69, 1978.

35. Rosen PP, Kosloff C, Lieberman PH et al. Lobular carcinoma in situ of the breast: Detailed analysis of 99 patients with average follow-up of 24 years. *Am J Surg Pathol* 2:225–51, 1978.

Chapter 6

1. Taubes G. Epidemiology faces its limits. *Science* 269: 164–69, 1995.

2. Gardner MJ and Altman DG. *Statistics with Confidence. British Medical Journal,* 1989.

3. Taubes G. Ibid.

4. Colditz, GA, Stampfer MJ, Willett WC et al. Prospective study of estrogen replacement therapy and risk of breast cancer in postmenopausal women. *JAMA* 264:2648–53, 1990.

5. Brinton, LA, Hoover R, and Fraumeni JF. Menopausal oestrogens and breast cancer risk: An expanded case-control study. *Br J of Cancer* 54:825–32, 1986.

6. Palmer JR, Rosenberg L, Clark EA et al. Breast cancer risk after estrogen replacement therapy: Results from the Toronto breast cancer study. *Am J Epidemiol* 134:1386–95. 1991.

7. Stanford, JL, Weiss NS, Voigt LF et al. Combined estrogen and progestin hormone replacement therapy in relation to risk of breast cancer in middle-aged women. *JAMA* 274:137–42, 1995.

8. Colditz GA, Stampfer MJ et al. Ibid.

9. Colditz, GA, Hankinson SE, Hunter DJ et al. The use of estrogens and progestins and the risk of breast cancer in postmenopausal women. *New Engl J Med* 332:1589–93, 1995.

10. Taubes G. Ibid.

11. Collaborative Group on Hormonal Factors in Breast Cancer. Breast cancer and hormone replacement therapy: Collaborative reanalysis of data from 51 epidemiological studies of 52,705 women with breast cancer and 108,411 women without breast cancer. *Lancet* 350:1047–59, 1997.

12. Brinton LA, Brogan DR, Coates RJ et al. Breast cancer risk among women under 55 years of age by joint effects of usage of oral contraceptives and hormone replacement therapy. *Menopause* 5:145–51, 1998; Kaufman DW et al. Ibid.; Palmer JR et al. Ibid.

13. Schairer C, Gail M, Byrne C et al. Estrogen replacement therapy and breast cancer survival in a large screening study, *J Natl Cancer Inst* 91:264–70, 2000.

14. Magnusson C, Holmberg L, Norden T et al. Prognostic characteristics in breast cancers after hormone replacement therapy. *Breast Cancer Research and Treatment* 38:325–34, 1996.

15. Ibid.; Bergkvist L, Adami H-O, Persson I et al. Prognosis after breast cancer diagnosis in women exposed to estrogen and estrogen progestogen. *Am J Epid* 130:221–28, 1989; Bonnier P, Romain S, Giacalone PL et al. Clinical and biologic prognostic factors in breast cancer diagnosed during postmenopausal hormone replacement therapy. *Obstet Gynecol* 85:11–17, 1995; Harding C, Knox WF, Faragher EB et al. Hormone replacement therapy and tumour grade in breast cancer: Prospective study in screening unit. *BMJ* 312:1646–47, 1996.

16. Strickland DM, Gambrell RD, Butzin CA et al. The relationship between breast cancer survival and prior postmenopausal estrogen use. *Obstet Gynecol* 80:400–4, 1992.

17. Bonnier P et al. Ibid.; Harding C et al. Ibid.

18. Grodstein F, Stampfer MJ, Colditz GA et al. Postmenopausal hormone therapy and mortality. *New Engl J Med* 336:1769–75, 1997.

19. Willis DB, Calle EE, Miracel-McMahill L et al. Estrogen replacement therapy and risk of fatal breast cancer in a prospective cohort of postmenopausal women in the United States. *Cancer Causes and Control* 7:449–57, 1996.

20. Sellers TA, Mink PJ, Cerhan JR et al. The role of hormone replacement therapy in the risk for breast cancer and total mortality in women with a family history of breast cancer. *Ann Intern Med* 127:973–80, 1997.

21. Eden JA, Bush T, Nand S et al. A case-control study of combined continuous estrogen-progestin replacement therapy among women with a personal history of breast cancer. *Menopause* 2:67–72, 1995.

22. Di Saia P, Grosen E, Kurosaki T et al. Hormone replacement therapy in breast cancer survivors: A cohort study. *Am J Ob Gyn* 174:1494–98, 1996; Vassilopoulou-Sellin R, Theriault R, Klein MJ. Estrogen replacement therapy in women with prior diagnosis and treatment for breast cancer. *Gynecol Oncol* 65:89–93, 1997; Guidozzi F. Estrogen replacement therapy in breast cancer survivors. *Int J Gynaecol Obstet* 64:59–63, 1999.

23. Vassilopoulou-Sellin R, Asmar L, Hortobagyi GN et al. Estrogen replacement therapy after localized breast cancer: Clinical outcome of 319 women followed prospectively. *J Clin Oncol* 17:1482–87, 1999.

24. *CA—A Cancer Journal for Clinicians. A Journal of the American Cancer Society* 50:21,23, 2000.

25. Phillips KA, Glendon, G, Knight JA. Putting the risk of breast cancer in perspective. *New Engl J Med* 340:141–44, 1999.

26. Ross, RK, Paganini-Hill A, Mack TM et al. Menopausal oestrogen therapy and protection from death from ischaemic heart disease. *Lancet*:858–60, 1981; Bush, TL, Barrett-Connor E, Cowan LD et al. Cardiovascular mortality and non-contraceptive use of estrogen in women: Results from the Lipid Research Clinics Program Follow-up Study. *Circulation* 75:1102–9, 1987.

27. Hulley S, Grady D, Bush T et al. Randomized trial of estrogen plus progestin for secondary prevention of coronary heart disease in postmenopausal women. *JAMA* 280:605–13, 1998.

28. Speroff L, Bush T, Clarkson TB et al. Hormone therapy and heart health in postmenopausal women. *Contemp Ob/Gyn* (Suppl.) November 1999. Oregon Health Sciences University:1–26.

Chapter 7

1. LaVecchia C, Negri E, Bruzzi P et al. The role of age at menarche and at menopause on breast cancer risk. Combined evidence from four case-control studies. *Ann Oncol* 3:625–29, 1992.

2. Brinton LA, Hoover R, Fraumeni JF. Interaction of familial and hormonal risk factors for breast cancer. *JNCI* 69:817–22, 1982; Sellers TA, Kushi LH, Potter JD. Effect of family history, body-fat distribution, and reproductive factors on the risk of postmenopausal breast cancer. *New Engl J Med* 326:1323–29, 1992; Andrieu N, Clavel F, Auquiet A et al. Variations in the risk of breast cancer associated with a family history of breast cancer according to age at onset and reproductive factors. *J Clin Epidemiol* 46:973–80, 1993.

3. Anderson DE and Badzioch MD. Combined effect of family history and reproductive factors on breast cancer risk. *Cancer* 63:349–53, 1989.

4. Weiss HA, Troisi R, Rossing MA et al. Fertility problems and breast cancer risk in young women: A case-control study in the United States. *Cancer Causes and Control* 9:331–39, 1998.

5. Anderson DE and Badzioch MD. Ibid.

6. Jernström H, Lerman C, Ghadirian P et al. Pregnancy and risk of early breast cancer in carriers of BRCA1 and BRCA2. *Lancet* 354:1846–50, 1999.

7. Rossing MA and Daling JR. Complexity of surveillance for cancer risk associated with in-vitro fertilisation. *Lancet* 354:1573–74, 1999.

8. Venn A, Watson L, Bruinsma F et al. Risk of cancer after use of fertility drugs with in-vitro fertilisation. *Lancet* 354:1586–90, 1999.

9. Newcomb PA, Storer BE, Longnecker MP et al. Lactation and a reduced risk of premenopausal breast cancer. *NEJM* 330:81–87, 1994.

10. Siskind V, Schofield F, Rice D, Bain C. Breast cancer and breast-feeding: Results from an Australian case-control study. *Am J Epid* 130:229–36, 1989; London SJ, Colditz GA, Stampfer MJ et al. Lactation and risk of breast cancer in a cohort of U.S. women. *Am J Epid* 132:17–26, 1990; Yang CP, Weiss, NS, Band PR et al. History of lactation and breast cancer risk. *Am J Epid* 138:1050–56, 1993.

11. Yang CP et al. Ibid.

12. LaVecchia et al. Ibid.

13. Sellers TA et al. Ibid.

14. Wynder El, Reddy BS, Weisburger JH. Environmental dietary factors in colorectal cancer. *Cancer* 70 (Suppl): 1222–28, 1992.

15. Smith-Warner SA, Spiegelman D, Yaun S-S et al. Alcohol and breast cancer in women: A pooled analysis of cohort studies. *JAMA* 279:535–40, 1998.

16. Willett WC, Stampfer MJ, Colditz, GA et al. Moderate alcohol consumption and the risk of breast cancer. *New Engl J Med* 316:1174–80, 1987.

17. Zhang Y, Kreger BE, Dorgan JF et al. Alcohol consumption and risk of breast cancer: The Framingham Study revisited. *Am J Epid* 149:93–101, 1999.

18. Smith-Warner SA, Spiegelman D, Yaun S-S et al. Ibid.

19. Collaborative Group on Hormonal Factors in Breast Cancer. Breast cancer and hormonal contraceptives: Collaborative reanalysis of individual data on 53,297 women with breast cancer and 100,239 women without breast cancer from 54 epidemiological studies. *Lancet* 347:1713–27, 1996.

20. Schonborn I, Nischan P, Ebeling K. Oral contraceptive use and the prognosis of breast cancer. *Breast Cancer Res Treat* 30(3):283–92, 1994; Beral V, Hermon C, Kay C et al. Mortality associated with oral contraceptive use: 25-year follow-up of cohort of 46,000 women from Royal College of General Practitioners' oral contraceptive study. *BMJ* 318:96–100, 1999.

21. Stanford JL, Brinton LA, Hoover RN. Oral contraceptives and breast cancer: Results from an expanded case-control study. *Br J Cancer* 60:375–81, 1989; Romieu I, Willett WC, Colditz GA et al. Prospective study of oral contraceptive use and risk of breast cancer in women. *J Natl Cancer Inst* 81:1313–21, 1989; White E, Malone KE, Weiss NS et al. Breast cancer among young U.S. women in relation to oral contraceptive use. *JNCI* 86:505–14, 1994.

22. Murray PP, Stadel BV, Schlesselman JJ. Oral contraceptive use in women with a family history of breast cancer. *Obstet Gynecol* 73:977–83, 1989; White E et al. Ibid.

23. Magnusson C, Colditz GA, Rosner B et al. Association of family history and other risk factors with breast cancer risk (Sweden). *Cancer Causes and Control* 9:259–67, 1998.

24. Kay CR and Hannaford PC. Breast cancer and the pill: A further report from the Royal College of General Practitioners' oral contraceptive study. *Br J Cancer* 58:675–80, 1988.

25. Olsson H, Borg A, Ferno M, Moller TR, Ranstam J. Early oral contraceptive use and premenopausal breast cancer: A review of studies performed in southern Sweden. *Cancer Detect Prev* 15:265–71, 1991.

Concluding Comments about Part II

1. Braddock CH, Edwards, KA, Hasenberg NM et al. Informed decision making in outpatient practice: Time to get back to basics. *JAMA* 282:2313–20, 1999.

2. Logan RL and Scott PJ. Uncertainty in clinical practice: Implications for quality and costs of health care. *Lancet* 347:5695–98, 1996.

Chapter 8

1. Braddock CH, Edwards, KA, Hasenberg NM et al. Informed decision making in outpatient practice: Time to get back to basics. *JAMA* 282:2313–20, 1999.

2. Ibid.

3. Kalet A, Roberts JC, Fletcher R. How do physicians talk with their patients about risks? *J Gen Intern Med* 9:402–4, 1994.

4. Dawes RM, Faust D, Meehl PE. Clinical versus actuarial judgment. *Science* 243:1668–74, 1989.

Chapter 9

1. Richards MPM, Hallowell N, Green JM. Counseling families with hereditary breast and ovarian cancer: A psychosocial perspective. *J Genet Counsel* 4:219–33, 1995.

2. Gail MH, Brinton LA, Byar P et al. Projecting individualized probabilities of developing breast cancer for white females who are being examined annually. *J Natl Cancer Inst* 81:1879–86, 1989; Claus EB, Risch N, Thompson D. Autosomal dominant inheritance of early-onset breast cancer: Implications for risk prediction. *Cancer* 73:645–51, 1994.

3. Spiegelman D, Colditz GA, Hunter D et al. Validation of the Gail et al. model for predicting individual breast cancer risk. *J Natl Cancer Inst* 86:600–7, 1994.

4. Stephenson J. Genetic test information fears unfounded. *JAMA* 282:2197–98, 1999.

Chapter 10

1. Weinstein ND. What does it mean to understand a risk? Evaluating risk comprehension. *Monogr Natl Cancer Inst* 25:15–20, 1999.

2. Tabar L, Duffy SW, Vitak B et al. The natural history of breast carcinoma. *Cancer* 86:449–62, 1999.

3. Hindle WH, Davis L, Wright D. Clinical value of mammography for symptomatic women 35 years of age and younger. *Am J Obstet Gynecol* 180:1484–90, 1999.

4. Joensuu H, Pylkkanen L, Toikkanen S. Late mortality from T1N0M0 breast carcinoma. *Cancer* 85:2183–89, 1999.

5. Stephenson J. Experts debate drugs for healthy women with breast cancer risk. *JAMA* 282:117–18, 1999.

6. Borgen PI, Hill ADK, Tran KN et al. Patient regrets after bilateral prophylactic mastectomy. *Ann Surg Oncol* 5:603–6, 1998.

7. Hartmann LC, Schaid DJ, Woods JE et al. Efficacy of bilateral prophylactic mastectomy in women with a family history of breast cancer. *New Engl J Med* 340:77–84, 1999.

8. Fisher B, Costantino JP, Wickerham DL et al. Tamoxifen for prevention of breast cancer: Report of the national surgical adjuvant breast and bowel project P-1 study. *J Natl Cancer Inst* 90:1371–88, 1998.

9. Cummings SR, Eckert S, Krueger KA et al. The effect of raloxifene on risk of breast cancer in postmenopausal women. *JAMA* 281:2189–97, 1999.

10. Ries LAG, Kosary CL, Hankey BF et al., eds. *SEER Cancer Statistics Review,* 1973–1996, National Cancer Institute, Bethesda, Md., 1999.

11. Piver MS, Jishi MF, Tsukada Y et al. Primary peritoneal carcinoma after prophylactic oophorectomy in women with a family history of ovarian cancer. *Cancer* 71:2751–55, 1993.

Chapter 11

1. Goleman D. *Vital Lies, Simple Truths: The Psychology of Self-Deception.* New York, Simon & Schuster, 1985, pp. 22, 24.

2. Macy J. *World As Lover, World As Self.* Berkeley, Parallax Press, 1991, p. 15.

3. Chodron, P. *When Things Fall Apart.* Boston, Shambhala, 1997.

4. Kaufman, BN. *Happiness Is a Choice.* New York, Ballantine Books, 1994.

Index

About the Author

PATRICIA T. KELLY, PH.D., is a medical geneticist who specializes in cancer risk assessment and counseling. A diplomate of the American Board of Medical Genetics and a founding fellow of the American College of Medical Genetics, Kelly lives in Berkeley, California.